GERMAN CANCER BREAKTHROUGH

Your Guide to Top German Alternative Clinics

Germany's cancer doctors lead the world — and Americans "in the know" go there to get well!

By Andrew Scholberg

D1261921

German Cancer Breakthrough
Your Guide to Top German Alternative Clinics

By Andrew Scholberg

Published by Online Publishing & Marketing, LLC

A Publication from *Cancer Defeated!*

IMPORTANT CAUTION:

By reading this special report you are demonstrating an interest in maintaining good and vigorous health.

This report suggests ways you can do that, but – as with anything in medicine – there are no guarantees.

You must check with private, professional medical advisors to assess whether the suggestions in this report are appropriate for you. And please note, the contents of this report may be considered controversial by the medical community at large.

The author, editors and publishers of this report are not doctors or professional health caregivers. They have relied on information from people who are. The information in this report is not meant to replace the attention or advice of physicians or other healthcare professionals. Nothing contained in this report is meant to constitute personal medical advice for any particular individual.

Every reader who wishes to begin any dietary, drug, exercise or other lifestyle changes intended to treat a specific disease or health condition should first get the advice of a qualified health care professional.

No alternative OR mainstream cancer treatment can boast a one hundred percent record of success. Far from it. There is ALWAYS some risk involved in any cancer treatment. The author, editors, and publishers of this report are not responsible for any adverse effects or results from the use of any of the suggestions, preparations or procedures described in this report. As with any medical treatment, results of the treatments described in this report will vary from one person to another.

PLEASE DO NOT USE THIS REPORT IF YOU ARE NOT WILLING TO ASSUME THE RISK.

The author reports here the results of a vast array of treatments and research as well as the personal experiences of individual patients, healthcare professionals and caregivers. In most cases the author was not present himself to witness the events described but relied in good faith on the accounts of the people who were.

ISBN 978-1-5323-2979-1

Printed in the United States of America

About the Author

Andrew Scholberg is a freelance writer living in Florida and a devotee of alternative medicine. With cancer activist Frank Cousineau, he co-authored two Special Reports, *America's Best Cancer Doctors and Their Secrets* and *Amish Cancer Secret.* He was the defendant in a landmark First Amendment case before the Supreme Court. In his spare time, Andrew is an adventurous outdoorsman.

Table Of Contents

Chapter One

Germany may offer the world's best cancer cure

As the late best-selling author, physician, and medical maverick Dr. Robert Atkins, M.D., once said:

"There is not one, but many cures for cancer available. But they are all being systematically suppressed by the American Cancer Society, the National Cancer Institute, and the major oncology centers. They have too much of an interest in the status quo."

Well, there you have it. Cures for cancer are available, but you don't know about them because too much money is at stake for those who are profiting from the status quo. They want you to submit to the old-fashioned, harsh and obsolete cancer treatment methods.

It's a shame that effective cancer cures are so hard to find in America. But there's no conspiracy to suppress these cancer cures in Germany. German doctors at the best clinics routinely use these cures to help "terminal" cancer patients get rid of their cancer – including American patients who fly to Germany for treatment.

We Americans pride ourselves on being Number One. After all, we're the last remaining world superpower. We have the world's richest economy. We win the most gold medals at the Olympics. We were the world's pioneers in space exploration. We're the only country that has actually put men on the moon, not just once but six times.

And we have the world-famous Mayo Clinic and other top-notch medical centers. Many would say we have the best medical care *in the world*.

Why, then, are so many Americans from all walks of life – from movie stars to people who can't afford health insurance – going to Germany for cancer treatment and for other medical care?

Before I answer that question, let me give you the names of some celebrities who've benefited from German therapies:

- Ronald Reagan
- Liz Taylor
- Cher
- Suzanne Somers
- Roy of "Siegfried and Roy"
- Jack Cassidy (the bass player from the Jefferson Airplane rock group)
- George Hamilton
- Red Buttons and his wife Alicia

You've probably seen the late comedian and actor Red Buttons in many movies over the years: "The Poseidon Adventure," "The Longest Day," "Alice in Wonderland," etc. When Red's wife Alicia was diagnosed with cancer in 1972, her American doctors gave her terrible news. She had an advanced case of one of the most dreaded cancers: oral pharyngeal cancer.

"Hopeless" patient lives 29 more years

Surgery for this kind of cancer leaves the patient with a disfigured face. For example, the late film critic Roger Ebert came down with oral cancer, and his American doctors performed drastic surgery on him. Sadly, the surgery left him severely disfigured and unable to speak during his final years.

The doctors told Alicia Buttons that her cancer was hopeless and terminal. They said, "With luck, you might be able to live a year."

But Red and his wife didn't take that American doctor's death sentence as the gospel truth. Instead, Red took his wife to Germany for mild, gentle alternative treatments that are non-toxic. And she lived for 29 more years.

Maybe you remember about what happened to Roy Horn of "Siegfried and Roy" on October 3, 2003. Apparently Roy stumbled or had some kind of seizure on stage. The white tiger, which loved Roy as his master, tried to come to his master's aid. And so the tiger picked Roy up by the neck as a mother cat picks up her kittens.

But people don't have the same kind of loose skin in the back of the neck that all cats do. So this bite caused severe damage.

Many people believed Roy's career was over. He was making hardly any improvement in American hospitals. So in June, 2005, he went to a clinic in Germany for alternative treatments. By May, 2007, Roy was testing out his new Mercedes at Little Bavaria. He announced to the public, "Look at me now – I am back, better than ever."

Following the devastating tiger attack, who would have ever thought that Roy would be back "better than ever" – in his own words?

Suzanne Somers chooses little-known German therapy

In 2001, actress Suzanne Somers got breast cancer at age 54, and she had surgery and radiation. Her American doctors strongly recommended that she follow up these treatments with chemo. They were aghast when Suzanne said no to their chemo and instead used mistletoe injections – a German therapy. The German therapy was successful.

All of the top cancer doctors in Germany use mistletoe therapy to boost their patients' immune systems.

Jennifer Lopez helped her aunt whip cancer in Germany

When Jennifer Lopez's aunt was losing her battle against ovarian cancer in a New York hospital, Jennifer paid for her treatment at one of Germany's finest cancer clinics. The aunt thanked her for helping her get "the best treatment possible" and described her experience at the clinic as "enlightening."

The treatments the aunt received in Germany were mild and healing. They weren't grueling and harsh like the American-style treatments that cause side effects such as baldness, nausea, violent retching, and loss of skin color.

The popular singer Cher of "Sonny & Cher" fame regularly goes to Germany for health tune-ups.

The brazen hypocrisy of the American cancer establishment

Let me tell you something you may find odd. Executives at organizations such as the American Cancer Society and agencies such as the U.S. Food and Drug Administration (FDA) strongly recommend that *you* undergo the traditional American treatment when *you* get cancer. So you'd think they'd practice what they preach when *they* get cancer, right?

Well, you're in for a surprise.

Back in 1987 a man named Jeff Harsh, who was working on a video documentary, interviewed one of Germany's top cancer physicians, Dr. Hans Nieper, M.D. (1928-1998). Dr. Nieper helped his patients, including Ronald Reagan, get rid of cancer by using alternative methods the FDA forbids in America. One of Dr. Nieper's forbidden methods was the natural substance called laetrile, which is derived from apricot seeds.

In the interview, Dr. Nieper said, "President Reagan is a very nice man," having treated him for cancer in July of 1983.

Dr. Neiper added, "You wouldn't believe how many FDA officials or relatives or acquaintances of FDA officials come to see me as patients in Hanover. You wouldn't believe this – or directors of the American Medical Association (AMA), or American Cancer Society (ACS), or the presidents of orthodox cancer institutes. That's the fact."

Well, there you have it. The wealthy executives who run the ACS, the FDA, and the AMA beat the drum for American-style cancer treatments that they recommend for *you* and your loved ones. But when *they* get cancer, well, that's different. Many of them head for Germany.

It's not just the rich and famous who go to Germany for medical treatment. You'll be shocked at how affordable the German clinics are compared to the sky-high prices American hospitals charge. Even some Americans who can't afford medical insurance find they can afford *German* medical treatment.

Why do Americans from all walks of life go to Germany for medical treatment? Well, there are at least three reasons:

Reason Number One: American doctors say, "Nothing more can be done" – but German doctors offer a ray of hope

Probably the most common reason so many American cancer patients choose Germany is because their American doctors have told them, "Nothing more can be done. You have no hope. You have only three months to live. Get your affairs in order."

American doctors are wrong to tell their patients, "Nothing more can be done." Instead, they should say, "We don't know of anything more that can be done." Doctors in Germany know more than a dozen other therapies that can be done. And the good news is that these German therapies are effective and non-toxic. What's more, they're amazingly inexpensive in comparison to American treatments.

Here's a partial list of some of the best therapies that patients can use:

- Whole body hyperthermia
- Local hyperthermia
- Insulin potentiation therapy (IPT)
- Mistletoe therapy
- Fever therapy
- Vitamin C and selenium by IV drip
- Ozone therapy
- Oxygen therapy
- Magnetic-field therapy
- Homeopathic therapy
- Detoxification therapy
- Colonic hydrotherapy
- Enzyme therapy
- Nutritional support
- Counseling
- Spiritual support

German doctors have found that a combination of these therapies can work – even when some other doctor has written off the patient as "hopeless." And the many American patients who've gotten rid of their cancer in Germany will attest to that.

In stark contrast to the repressive situation in the USA, all of these advanced therapies have the approval of Germany's health ministry, and the German government has licensed the clinics.

In this book, I will describe the German therapies as best I can. But I'm a layman, not a doctor, and so my ability to describe the technical aspects of the treatments is limited. If you're looking for scholarly, technical explanations, I'll give you some references you can look up in medical libraries or on the Internet.

Unfortunately, the typical American doctor only learns one approach to cancer treatment in medical school: the "cut-burn-poison" approach. The American method of treating cancer focuses on surgery, radiation, and chemotherapy while ignoring the cause of the cancer and the natural therapies that can address the cause.

Let me be crystal clear about this: American doctors are not evil. They're not deliberately concealing vital information from their cancer patients. Most American doctors just don't know about alternative therapies. They apply what they learned in medical school. They assume that what they learned about cancer in medical school is all there is to know about it.

Wrong!

Patients shouldn't die from their *treatments*!

Tragically, American medicine has an abysmal record in treating cancer. Despite what you hear about progress and "new discoveries," mainstream American cancer treatment today isn't much different than the cut-burn-poison treatments of 50 years ago. And the worst part of these treatments is that they're often as hard on the patient as they are on the cancer. Yes, the radiation and chemo sometimes kill off the cancer cells, but the same radiation and chemo often destroys the patient's immune system. This can easily cause death.

American doctors might triumphantly declare, "We killed the cancer!" But what does that matter if the patient died from the toxic treatments?

Fortunately, the word is starting to reach many Americans that German doctors have achieved a real breakthrough in cancer treatment.

Should anyone be surprised that the Germans are arguably the finest cancer doctors in the world?

Let's face it: The Germans are noted for spectacular achievements. It was German rocket scientists in Russia who launched Sputnik, which inaugurated the space age. It was German rocket scientists in America who were essential to putting men on the moon.

Germans have made countless scientific and technical breakthroughs. Here are just a few:

- In 1714 Daniel Gabriel Fahrenheit invented the mercury thermometer.
- In 1885 Karl Benz (of Mercedes-Benz fame) built the first practical car run by internal combustion, and Gottlieb Daimler invented his landmark gasoline engine.
- Rudolf Diesel invented the engine named for him
- In 1899 Felix Hoffman was the first to synthesize a medically useful form of aspirin. Bayer, a German company, manufactured Hoffman's new product.
- In 1916 Albert Einstein announced his general theory of relativity

Today the Germans make some of the world's finest cars and the finest optical products. In fact, Germany is still a top exporter of high-quality manufactured products while the United States, sadly, has slipped behind.

Is it any wonder that in cancer treatment, German doctors leave most American cancer doctors in the dust?

Reason #2: It costs $800,000 to *die* of cancer in America!

Surprisingly, the second reason Americans go to Germany for cancer treatment is because some people can't afford the American cancer treatments. It can easily cost $800,000 to die of cancer in the USA. By contrast, an American cancer patient can go to Germany for a three-week course of treatment for the price of a Honda Accord.

What if someone can't afford health insurance? How could he or she possibly afford a six-figure medical bill? Who has hundreds of thousands of dollars just sitting in their bank account? Not many.

During a visit to one of the German cancer clinics I met Franko, a patient from Key West, Florida. Franko had no health insurance, but he was able to afford the mild but effective German-style cancer treatments. Franko told me the cost of his cancer treatment in Germany was worth it. He said, "Is your life worth a new Honda?"

Reason Number Three: Gentle treatments that are more effective

The third reason Americans go to Germany for cancer treatment is because they prefer the mild but effective treatments available there. The German cancer doctors I interviewed avoid surgery and radiation unless it's absolutely necessary. And *if* they give any chemotherapy, it's a fraction of the dose American doctors give.

In this book I'm going to take you on a virtual tour of the most outstanding cancer treatment centers in Germany, Switzerland, and Austria. You'll learn all about the German-style cancer treatments, and you'll meet some of the most brilliant minds in medicine: doctors who routinely save the lives of cancer patients whom American doctors have declared "hopeless" and "terminal."

You'll also meet American patients as well as some English-speaking foreign patients. Each of them has a unique story, and I'm eager to tell you these stories.

I visited one clinic in Munich that I can't recommend for Americans because the personnel in that clinic don't speak English fluently. The Munich clinic is set up for the local cancer patients. Americans and others who don't speak German would feel out of place in that clinic.

One of the things that surprised me is that none of the clinics looked or smelled like a hospital. Rather, the atmosphere was cheerful, friendly, and warm. The German clinics seemed more like hotels or bed & breakfasts. Patients wear their own clothes at the German clinics – not those flimsy hospital gowns that leave your backside exposed.

"Bad" doesn't mean the opposite of good!

Some of the most outstanding clinics are located in Bad Mergentheim, Bad Salzhausen, Bad Bergzabern, and Bad Aibling. Now, you may be wondering why some of these towns begin with the word "Bad." It doesn't mean that these towns are "bad." On the contrary; they're wonderful. The German word "Bad" (pronounced "Bahd") means bath. In other words, these are spa towns. Each town has mineralized springs that are said to have healing, curative properties. Health seekers have sought out these springs for centuries – going back to Roman times.

I'll tell you what you need to know about each clinic – treatments, costs, and practical considerations – as well as the contact information.

You can benefit from German therapies in the comfort of your home

Perhaps the most important chapter in this book is the one entitled "Cancer Dilemma: Do you swat mosquitoes or drain the swamp?" In other words, do you just treat the symptoms of cancer, or do you get at the root of the problem so it doesn't come back?

Let's say you've gone to one of the German clinics I recommend, and you've gotten rid of your cancer. You've come home cancer free. Now what?

Although I'm not a doctor, I've visited 43 of the top holistic, integrative cancer clinics in the United States, Mexico, Switzerland, Austria, and Germany. I've interviewed the doctors at these clinics. I've interviewed their patients. In short, I've seen what works and what doesn't work.

To put the odds in your favor, you need to make permanent lifestyle changes. You don't want to spend the rest of your life returning to doctors each time cancer returns. That's like "swatting mosquitoes." Rather, the goal is to get rid of cancer *for good*. And to accomplish that goal, you have to "drain the swamp." That requires permanent changes in your life.

Changing your eating plan is especially important. The typical American diet, which is high in both sugar and red meat, will likely cause the cancer to return with a vengeance. The doctors I interviewed describe eating plans you can use for the rest of your life. You'll be able to eat meals that are tasty and nourishing but unfriendly and unwelcoming toward cancer.

If excess stress has caused or contributed to your cancer, you need to learn how to manage the stress so it doesn't tear down your immune system.

A regular program of detoxification is essential, too. All of the German clinics I visited understand the importance of colonic hydrotherapy. This is something you can do wherever you live. The services of a professional colonic hydrotherapist are inexpensive. With the right equipment, you can even do colonic hydrotherapy at home.

Magnetic field therapy is another effective treatment you can do at home. This therapy wakes up your immune system and tells it to get busy. You can own the very same sophisticated magnetic field machine the German cancer clinics use. It costs about as much as a 15-year-old car with high miles.

Some German cancer clinics put their patients on the magnetic-field therapy machine *every day* for 15 minutes because it's such an effective immune system booster. Why should this amazing therapy stop when you come home from Germany? It doesn't have to.

We recommend, however, that you seek the advice of a competent medical authority before using magnetic field therapy or any of the other therapies mentioned in this book.

Intravenous vitamin C therapy can also continue at home, and I'll tell you how to find a doctor willing to give you this therapy. A man from Oklahoma who got rid of a nasty form of brain cancer in Germany over five years ago gets IV vitamin C therapy once a month right here in America. If this therapy has helped him keep cancer at bay, it could help you, too.

After all, the goal isn't just to get rid of cancer but to keep it away *for good*.

Chapter Two

Dr. Holgar Wehner's Gisunt Klinik in Wilhelmshaven

"There are no untreatable patients"

Most of the top cancer clinics in Germany are reasonably close to Frankfurt or Munich. But the Gisunt Klinik, founded by Dr. Holgar Wehner, M.D., one of Germany's top cancer doctors, is located in the far northwestern corner of Germany in the coastal town of Wilhelmshaven.

When you think of Germany, it's unlikely that the image of an oceanside beach will come to mind. But if you stay at the Gisunt Klinik in Wilhelmshaven, you'll be right next to a UNESCO World Natural Heritage Site: the Lower Saxony Wadden Sea National Park with mile after mile of beaches along the North Sea. You'll also be under the care of a seasoned physician who has an impressive track record treating patients who have even the most difficult cancers.

For example, perhaps the toughest, deadliest, fastest-growing cancer is glioblastoma multiforme brain cancer. This is the kind of cancer that killed Senator Ted Kennedy. In America, it's considered a death sentence. Not so in Germany.

A desperate 30-year-old German woman, Margaret Krauss, was diagnosed with glioblastoma multiforme brain cancer and needed to beat the disease for the sake of her young daughter. Conventional doctors had already given her surgery and radiation, but to no avail.

In 1999 Margaret came to the Gisunt Klinik as a last resort, and put her life in Dr. Wehner's hands. In addition to other therapies, Dr. Wehner gave three sets of 12 hyperthermia treatments. After the third set, she was in complete remission. Margaret has been cancer free ever since then and is still alive today. Her case was so extraordinary that it was featured in a TV documentary.

Dr. Wehner has successfully treated three other patients with glioblastoma multiforme brain cancer as well. One of them, a man who started treatment at Gisunt in 2009, has passed his five-year cancer survival milestone and remains in complete remission to this day.

Dr. Wehner has become famous for using every form of hyperthermia – heat therapy – which he considers an essential part of holistic, integrative cancer treatment.

"Give me the power to induce fever, and I'll cure any disease"

Why is hyperthermia such an effective treatment? It's a form of heat therapy, which is nothing new. Five centuries before Christ, the father of medicine, Hippocrates, recognized the curative power of fevers. Another ancient Greek, Parmenides, said, "Give me the power to induce a fever, and I will cure any disease."

That's why Dr. Wehner says a fever shouldn't be suppressed as long as it's not life-threatening. Natural fevers train and strengthen the immune system and should generally be allowed to run their course.

Extreme hyperthermia kills cancer cells by the millions

During an "extreme" whole body hyperthermia treatment, the patient gets an artificial fever of 42 to 42.5 degrees Celsius for two hours. That's 107.6 to 108.5 degrees Fahrenheit! You might think that's dangerous, but it's not. You might think that a core temperature of 108.5 degrees Fahrenheit would cause brain damage, but it doesn't.

You see, at Gisunt the whole process of extreme hyperthermia is carefully monitored while the patient is under general anesthesia. Infrared heat, filtered through water, gently warms the layer of skin that contains blood. The heated blood circulates, and more blood is gently heated, until the desired core temperature is reached. To protect the brain from getting overheated, cold patches are placed on carotid arteries on both sides of the neck at more than 41.5 degrees Celsius. Dr. Wehner has vast experience administering extreme hyperthermia, and he knows how to do it with complete safety.

Dr. Wehner told me, "Research indicates that we need every tenth of a degree more than 42 Celsius. We have done over 2,000 treatments higher than 42. The maximum safe level is 42.5. at 42 degrees and up, we have tumor killing. The very lowest temperature that kills tumor cells is 41.5 (106.7 degrees Fahrenheit), but only when the pH goes down. When the pH is lower, tumor cells are more sensitive to hyperthermia. Then and only then can you kill tumor cells at 41.5.

"The patient is under deep intravenous anesthesia. The patient sleeps during the therapy. It's easy. There are no complications, and we're happy about that. The patient breathes spontaneously. We've never seen complications. The best protocol for extreme hyperthermia is 90 minutes higher than 41.5 degrees, 60 minutes higher than 41.8, and 30 minutes higher than 42 degrees. This is the standard protocol for the moment. We have success in late-stage cancer with 65 percent

responding well. Patients who reject chemo and use hyperthermia alone have also had good results. We also have documentation that extreme hyperthermia works for our glioblastoma multiforme brain cancer patients."

Of course, no clinic has a 100 percent success rate. Many patients have had their immune systems severely compromised by too much chemo or radiation before they seek treatment at a place like Gisunt. Sometimes patients wait too late to seek holistic, complementary therapy. But even in these cases, integrative treatment can relieve suffering and give the patient a better quality of life.

At the Gisunt Klinik, cancer patients can get all forms of hyperthermia:

- Whole body hyperthermia as described above
- Local hyperthermia in which heat penetrates deeply into a specific portion of the body to weaken or kill the tumor
- Transurethral local hyperthermia for prostate cancer, in which a catheter with a special heating device is painlessly inserted through the urethra into the prostate. Once inserted, the heat is applied to the prostate, cooking the cancer to death without harming the healthy tissue or causing discomfort to the patient. This procedure isn't just for prostate cancer but also treats prostatitis and benign prostate hyperplasia (BPH), which means enlarged prostate.
- Intraperitoneal hyperthermia for abdominal cancers. The peritoneal cavity is rinsed with a hyperthermal wash that may contain chemo. In cases of bladder cancer, the bladder can be rinsed with the same chemo-infused hyperthermal wash.

At Gisunt, patients are prepared for whole body hyperthermia with an application of oil on the skin followed by a specially prepared whirlpool bath. In 20 minutes Dr. Wehner can get the patient's core temperature up to the high plateau that kills tumor cells by the millions.

Dr. Wehner is well qualified to apply all forms of hyperthermia, considering that he's the president of the German Society of Hyperthermia.

No patient is considered untreatable!

Although no doctor can guarantee a successful outcome, Dr. Wehner is confident that he can help just about any patient. He says, "There are no untreatable patients." Patients who arrive in wheelchairs are often able to get up and *walk* out of the clinic when they go home.

Although Dr. Wehner is best known as a cancer doctor, he also treats other chronic conditions such as burn-out syndrome, fatigue syndrome, stress syndrome, metabolic diseases, circulation disorders, migraines, dizziness, tinnitus, hearing loss, fibromyalgia, psoriasis, colitis, Crohn's disease, asthma, and joint-, muscle-, and skeletal ailments.

While touring Gisunt I met a British patient's companion who had read my book *German Cancer Breakthrough* from cover to cover. She said, "I have this book. It's very good. You're the one who wrote it?" I said, "Yes, I'm Andrew Scholberg." She said, "Oh my goodness. It's so amazing that I've got your book. I have the Kindle version. It was invaluable. I can't believe that. I'm very glad. I'll tell my friend."

When I sat down to interview Dr. Wehner, I asked him to tell me his story. He told me he started out as a surgeon but changed to natural medicine to get better results. In 1985 he started using hyperthermia and has never looked back. One of his four children, a daughter, is now a medical doctor who did her dissertation on hyperthermia.

Dr. Wehner is well acquainted with Germany's top cancer doctors, including Dr. Friedrich Douwes, Dr. Friedrich Migeod, and Dr. Alexander Herzog. These collegial doctors are profiled in other chapters of this book: Dr. Douwes in the chapter about St. Georg Klinik, Dr. Migeod in the chapter about BioMed Klinik, and Dr. Herzog in the chapter about his Fachklinik.

Patients who seek cancer treatment at Gisunt should plan on a three-week stay. Dr. Wehner says that if a patient can only come for a week, "forget it." A week isn't enough time for the necessary treatments including detoxification, immune boosting therapies, oxygen therapy, mistletoe, and hyperthermia with low-dose chemo.

Patients from around the world come to Gisunt

Patients come to the Gisunt Klinik from as far away as Australia, Africa, Korea, and the United Arab Emirates. When I toured Gisunt, Dr. Wehner was treating one patient from Ghana, three from the United Kingdom, one from America, and the rest from Germany. Gisunt has a friendly atmosphere, like a family, and you're likely to meet some interesting people there.

On the wall of Dr. Wehner's office is the 2,500-year-old Oath of Hippocrates, which he took upon graduating from medical school. He has the heart of a healer and a warm and cheerful personality. He told me, "I love my work. When you have good results, the patient is happy, and we're happy. It's very positive."

Dr. Wehner said that his location on the North Sea is a disadvantage because many patients prefer a clinic that's closer to Frankfurt or Munich. Nevertheless, the patients who make the extra effort to travel to his clinic are happy with their choice.

One patient, a lady from the United Kingdom, was inclined to choose a different clinic after reading an earlier edition of this book. But her husband called all of the clinics in my book, and Gisunt was the only one where he was able to speak on the phone with a doctor, so he persuaded his wife to go to Gisunt. Her ovarian cancer is now under control, thanks to Dr. Wehner.

Recreational activities keep cancer patients busy

Gisunt encourages exercise and offers its patients lots of activities. You can go Nordic Walking in parks or by the sea. If you enjoy cultural and artistic events, Gisunt can help you attend local performances. Patients enjoy visiting the local museums and shops. You can even take a boat to one of the beautiful East Frisian islands or visit Jever, the historic castle town. Dr. Wehner believes that activities like these are important because cancer patients benefit greatly when they're active, happy, smile often, and manage their stress.

Indeed, Dr. Wehner told me, "What's needed is an integrative concept that addresses the mind, soul, and body." (The German word "Gisunt" means healthy. As you may have guessed, this word is related to "Gesundheit," which is commonly said even in certain parts of America to wish good health to someone who has just sneezed. For example, I often heard "Gesundheit" after someone sneezed when I was growing up in Minneapolis.)

Wilhelmshaven is certainly a healthy location. The air is as clean as you'll find anywhere in Germany because the prevailing winds come across the sea from the northwest, where there's no industry. Filling the lungs with fresh air while exercising gives cancer patients and others a big health boost. Dr. Wehner increases this boost with a special form of oxygen therapy known as EWOT, which stands for Exercise With Oxygen Therapy. In EWOT, the patient inhales pressurized oxygen through a mask for 20 minutes and then spends 10 minutes pedaling a stationary bicycle or walking stairs, then another 20 minutes of inhaling pressurized oxygen through the mask, and another 10 minutes of exercise.

Patients do EWOT for two hours a day, every day for 18 days. Dr. Wehner says it helps overcome fatigue syndrome, and hyperoxygenation makes the tissues more sensitive for extreme hyperthermia.

Dr. Wehner also offers light therapy. Patients are encouraged to relax and read something next to a lighting device that kicks out 17,500 lux, which is a unit of luminance. Dr. Wehner told me this therapy is good for patients who are tired, and it also has a positive effect against depression.

The cost of treatment at Gisunt

Cancer treatment lasting three weeks, including extreme hyperthermia sessions, costs about 10,000 Euros per week: 30,000 Euros total. Compared to conventional American treatments, 30,000 Euros is a bargain. Before committing to treatment at Gisunt, be sure to get an estimated cost of the proposed treatment plan because prices change, and some treatments may cost extra.

Accommodations at Gisunt Klinik are easy. Dr. Wehner can accommodate inpatients, and for outpatients there's a lovely hotel across the street next to a park. For patients who want to rent a car there are no traffic problems, and plenty of parking is available. Bicycle riding is easy because there are no hills in town.

How to get to the Gisunt Klinik

The closest airport is Bremen, which is an hour's drive from the Gisunt Klinik. Bremen is a 45 minute flight from Amsterdam. You can also fly to Frankfurt and easily take a connecting flight to Bremen. When you arrive in Bremen, a driver from Gisunt will meet you at the airport and drive you to your destination in the comfort of a spacious van. A huge, rustic windmill that's almost 200 years old is right next to the Gisunt Klinik. Gisunt's street, Mühlenweg, means "Mill Way."

Contact information:

Dr. Holgar Wehner, Medical Director

Gisunt Klinik for Integrative Medicine
Mühlenweg 144
D - 26384 Wilhelmshaven
Germany

e-mail: info@gisunt.de

Website: www.gisunt-klinik.de

Phone: 011-49-4421-77414-0

Fax: 011-49-4421-77414-10

Chapter Three

Lothar Hirneise's 3E Center near Stuttgart

Lothar Hirneise and his colleague Klaus Pertl co-founded and co-direct one of the most unusual cancer centers in Germany. Neither of them is a physician. What they've created is a unique place for people with cancer – a "seminar house" – that has achieved stunning, extraordinary results for cancer patients who'd been told their condition was "terminal."

To prove the results of their center, Lothar did a prospective study of 67 terminal cancer patients who went through his five-week program. At the time of their admission, all of the patients had written documentation from their doctors that their life expectancy was six months on average: some were given just a few weeks to live, and a few were given a year at most. These patients were at the end of their rope. They had all undergone some conventional therapy, and their conventional doctors had nothing to offer them except palliative care, having declared them "terminal." They all came to the 3E Center as a last resort.

At the end of 23 months, all 67 patients should have been dead, according to what their doctors had predicted in writing. But at the end of 23 months over half of the patients in the study were still alive: 36 of the 67 who started! That should have been front-page news worldwide.

Here's the breakdown. At the end of the study, seven patients with multiple metastases and one patient with inoperable glioblastoma brain cancer (the deadliest kind!) were tumor free. Ten more patients also became tumor free, but it took longer than 23 months.

Other surviving patients achieved a state of stable disease. In other words, they still had their tumors, but the tumors were inactive – not causing any problems. Just as many people live next to an inactive volcano without problems, so many patients can enjoy an excellent quality of life for decades in a state of stable disease with inactive tumors.

Lothar told me, "No one can say that 'they really didn't have cancer' or that it was 'luck' or 'spontaneous remission.' There was nothing spontaneous about it. It was healing. It took hard work."

A radiologist who examined Lothar's patients with inactive tumors told him, "I don't understand what you're doing. I don't understand why the PET scans of your patients look different from the other patients' PET scans." He has never seen any PET scans from patients of conventional doctors that show *totally inactive tumors*. Lothar attributes it to the Budwig diet. But his patients aren't too interested in the explanation because they're just happy to be healthy and living a normal life.

Another thing that's remarkable about Lothar's study is that he achieved such success without any hyperthermia, which is a key treatment at all of the other cancer clinics I visited in Germany, Austria, and Switzerland.

Lothar's study proves how foolish it is for any doctor to predict how much time a cancer patient has. Cancer has become the No. 1 fear for many people, as infectious diseases such as TB and smallpox were in past times. That's why many believe a cancer diagnosis means their life is over, and they readily believe a doctor who tells them they should get their affairs in order because they have "three months" or "six months" to live.

To find out the secret of the 3E Center's success, I interviewed Lothar for more than three hours, during which he explained the three essential aspects of his program: (1) the Johanna Budwig anti-cancer eating plan, (2) detoxification, and (3) counseling (mind-body medicine).

With true German hospitality, when I met Lothar he offered me a dessert, which I readily accepted. After I'd eaten it, he asked me if I'd tasted the flax oil. I said no. I had just eaten Johanna Budwig's famous mixture of flax oil, milk, and quark blended with some fruit. Quark, which is common in Europe, is virtually the same as cottage cheese.

The lifesaving discoveries of the legendary Dr. Budwig

Lothar became a close friend and colleague of Dr. Johanna Budwig (1908-2003), who authorized him to promote and teach her anti-cancer protocol, which includes her famous mixture of flax oil, cottage cheese, and milk. The strict and correct application of the Budwig protocol makes the 3E Center unique. Lothar is firmly convinced that the Budwig potocol is the main reason why he gets such outstanding results for cancer patients.

I asked Lothar to give me a layman's explanation of Dr. Budwig's reasoning behind the flax oil/cottage cheese combination. He said, "You want to create a lipoprotein – a mixture of fat and protein. And you want to make the fat *water soluble*. That's the whole idea. You could eat the fat and protein separately, but it wouldn't work. You have to thoroughly mix the two before eating it. Then the energy – that is, the electrons stored in the flax oil – is changed and becomes water soluble so it can go everywhere in your tissues and blood *without first having to go through the liver*. If it had to go through the liver first, it would lose energy.

"Dr. Budwig's whole idea was to quickly bring energy to the body. Cancer patients have two main problems: (1) an energy problem and (2) a cell membrane problem. A cell membrane is mostly fat and phosphate. The Budwig mixture brings good fat back to the cell membrane so it works as it should. A healthy cell membrane has a tension of -70 to -90 millivolts in electricity. But it's -60, -40, or lower in cancer cells. Our main strategy to fix that is the Budwig eating plan, but we also have some machines to help bring the proper tension back into the cell membrane."

Dr. Budwig, wanting to bring more energy to the cancer patient's body, asked the question: Where can you find the most electrons? In other words, what food has the most energy? When she found the extraordinary energy level in fresh flax oil, her search was over. Lothar explained that flax oil is the *only known food* containing a carbon chain with *three* double bonds. But Dr. Budwig understood that just drinking the flax oil wouldn't work because the oil would have to go through the stomach, liver, and colon. She wanted to find a way to get the energy directly into the blood *fast*! Blending the fresh flax oil with quark (or cottage cheese) and milk proved to be the answer.

Budwig hated olive oil. She called it the most useless oil in the world because 90 percent of it has only one double bond. It bears repeating that flax oil has *three* double bonds.

Lothar also likes coconut oil, which is solid and, unlike many oils, can be heated to high temperatures without creating toxins. The benefit of eating coconut fat is that the fat doesn't have to go through the liver: your body absorbs it and uses it as a fast energy without burdening the liver. Coconut oil is widely available.

"*Never* eat margarine," cautioned Lothar. "It doesn't matter what the manufacturers are saying. They're lying. Eating it is like eating plastic."

The Budwig protocol is an anti-cancer eating plan, and the mixture of flax oil, cottage cheese, and milk is only a part of the overall plan. It's a vegetarian plan, which includes fresh-pressed juice. Lothar said, "Cancer patients have long protein chains, rubbish, in the body, and the enzymes in papaya juice help break down the protein chains." Patients usually get papaya juice every second day, and carrot juice on the other days.

Lothar said that raw sauerkraut contains a good kind of lactate that helps repair the colon. In fact, he calls sauerkraut "the queen of lactate." Each morning, patients at the center drink up to 200 milliliters (nearly seven ounces) of raw sauerkraut juice – another powerful remedy that's dirt cheap.

This is an important part of the Budwig eating plan. The way the good lactate in sauerkraut juice works, Lothar explained, is that it makes a connection with the "bad" lactate a tumor is producing (called racemate), and goes into the blood where it can then go into the liver. Once it enters the liver it produces the sugar that's needed for energy. Sauerkraut juice and baking soda baths get over 90 percent of the bad lactate out of the cancer patient's body and change the pH value of the blood, which normally is too high in cancer patients.

The lactate the tumor produces isn't the same at all because most of it remains stuck in the tissue, where it does no good whatsoever. Lothar said, "Raw sauerkraut juice gives the patient five to 10 to 15 times the energy that sauerkraut gives." He feels so strongly about the benefits of raw sauerkraut juice that, he remarked, it should be sold for $100 a bottle because then people might take it seriously.

Cheap solutions sometimes work better than expensive solutions. Low-tech sometimes beats high-tech.

Breakfast consists of the famous Budwig mixture of flax oil, cottage cheese, and milk, blended with some kind of fruit (but not bananas, which Lothar says are too sugary for cancer patients).

Here's the recipe for the mixture: 150 to 200 grams of cottage cheese plus 3 or 4 tablespoons of fresh, refrigerated flax oil plus half of that amount of whole milk (1.5 to 2 tablespoons). Thoroughly blend this basic mixture. After it's thoroughly blended, you can add berries or some other kind of fruit and blend everything together.

IMPORTANT: Don't try to blend everything all at once. Instead, blend the basic mixture first, and then if you add berries, hit the "blend" button again. Lothar says the very same recipe can also be used by healthy patients who want to prevent cancer and by patients whose cancer is in remission, to prevent it from coming back.

A good test of the mixture is that it should have no yellow color from the flax oil. If it does, the flax oil is probably oxidized (i.e. spoiled) and should be thrown out. Flax oil oxidizes easily, which is why it needs to be kept refrigerated.

The Budwig mixture must be completely water soluble. After eating it, you should be able to hold the bowl under running water to rinse it out. The Budwig mixture won't work if the flax oil or the cottage cheese are bad. Both must be fresh.

Lothar recommends *plain* flax oil. He frowns on flax oil with lignans and says flaxseed oil capsules are also bad.

I asked Lothar if it's necessary to let the basic mixture sit for five minutes before eating it, as I had heard. He replied that no waiting is necessary: once it's thoroughly blended, you can eat it right away.

For lunch, patients eat raw vegetarian food. Supper is a light combination of cooked vegetables and soup. The cooking is done slowly, and no microwave is on the property. Patients can have a no-sugar dessert. Lothar said, "Many hospitals say they have a good kitchen, but that's not always the case. For us, it's Job One!"

To make the food as delicious as it can be, the center employs two professional chefs who know the techniques for making food look and taste delicious. When they joined the clinic, they just needed some coaching about what they could and couldn't use to create culinary masterpieces that fit within the Budwig eating plan. For example, buckwheat normally doesn't taste good, but the center's chefs have a way of preparing it so that it's delicious. Lothar declared, "We could open a restaurant here. Our food is that good."

Avoiding carbs will starve cancer cells, right? Wrong

Some sugars are worse than others. Lothar said, "If you don't eat sugar, your liver will produce a substitute for sugar, but cancer cells also love this substitute. It's not easy to kill tumor cells by not eating *any* sugar. Patients can eat one gram of good carbs (non-starchy vegetables, for example) for every kilo of body weight."

Lothar believes it makes no sense to eat no carbohydrates at all: "The last thing you want to do is stay away from carbs, otherwise the liver has to work harder to produce ketones."

He has seen tremendous results with the Budwig eating plan, which allows some bread (but not much because it quickly converts to blood sugar in the body) and some potatoes but no noodles. Each patient gets the right portion, based on the patient's weight.

Why champagne can be good for cancer patients

I was startled when Lothar said, "We give the patients champagne." I'd never heard any such thing at a cancer clinic, but Lothar explained that Budwig had solid, scientific reasons for making champagne a part of the eating plan for most cancer patients.

Lothar explained, "Champagne is a double-fermented alcohol, so that when you drink it, it goes right into your blood stream, much faster than beer. Champagne also helps the colon because only double-fermented alcohol can kill bad bacteria in the gut. But the main reason we give champagne to cancer patients is to help pick up their energy. Another benefit of

champagne is that the sugar in the alcohol can't be absorbed by cancer cells.

"When you give champagne, you'll see little wonders. When a new patient arrives at our center hunched over from lack of energy, we give the patient two glasses of champagne in the morning or in the afternoon. It works very well." Lothar remarked that he and Budwig drank a lot of champagne together.

Budwig believed cancer is mainly a problem of energy. She said that if you bring more energy into the body than the cancer cells are absorbing, the cancer patient will survive. That's why Lothar uses a variety of ways to get as much energy into the body as possible. One of the most important ways is simply to be outside in the open air to absorb energy from the sun.

He said, "We encourage patients to be outside. If they can stay outside all day long, that's best. When they come in for lunch or dinner, they have to go for a walk outside afterward because we want the carbs to go to the muscles and not be stored in the liver. We send them out, appropriately dressed, even if it's raining or snowing. They have to walk or do some kind of physical activity.

"Even when you're outside after dark, you get cosmic waves from the sun. Of course, the sun's cosmic waves are stronger when the patient is outside during daylight hours."

The 3E Center's idyllic surroundings

Fortunately, the 3E Center is located out in the country, and the center's grounds and surrounding countryside are beautiful. There are apple trees by the outdoor patio area, and also an impressive circular deck by the center in front of the pond.

The center is built with all-natural, non-toxic materials only. Instead of carpeting, the floors are made of hardwood and stone. The lounge area is pleasant and peaceful – with no TV. The center believes patients should focus on themselves and get rid of stress through meditation and other therapies instead of getting bad news, negativity, and stress from the television.

The center consists of three buildings that are interconnected in a way that flows naturally for the way of life there. The dining room is the heart and soul of the center. A walkway leads from the dining room to the meditation area, where the counseling and various therapies take place. Another walkway leads from the meditation area to the living area. The whole complex is heated with geothermal energy, which is pollution free.

Although Lothar isn't a painter, he's good at drawing. He designed the paintings that decorate the center. After sketching out the painting he has in mind, he sends his sketch to China and pays a Chinese artist to do the actual painting. The resulting art is beautiful.

Lothar's story

I asked Lothar how he became interested in natural treatments for cancer. His story is fascinating. He worked as a nurse for three years, studied psychoanalysis for four years, and then worked for four years in psychotherapy. Altogether, he spent 12 years working in psychiatric and psychotherapy hospitals, which burned him out.

He decided to do something completely different and started a sports business selling boxing gloves and martial arts devices. His success was extraordinary, and he became a competitor to Everlast. He was a sponsor to the Olympic Games in Atlanta in 1996 and sold his company later that year. The company, Top Ten Boxing Gloves, still exists.

Having made sufficient money in business, Lothar didn't have to work for his daily bread and could have retired, but he was restless and not sure what to do with his life. Around that time a friend of his became seriously ill with testicular cancer and went through chemotherapy. Lothar attended a health fair with his friend Klaus Pertl and asked the author of *What Doctors Don't Tell You*, Lynne McTaggart, about cancer and alternative treatments. She urged him to attend a major alternative cancer conference in London the following month. She said, "Just come. I'll introduce you to the speakers and you can ask them what they would do for your friend."

Lothar flew to London for the three-day conference, during which his friend with testicular cancer died. He and his friend Klaus found it "interesting" to hear what those "crazy" people were saying. They started flying to clinics all over the world to find out what works and what doesn't work.

After founding an organization in Germany called People Against Cancer, Lothar came up with the idea to open a cancer center to help patients and to promote the Budwig protocol. His friend Klaus agreed to be the co-founder. Their 3E Center opened in 2006.

They work with two medical doctors, who regularly visit the center, plus up to three alternative practitioners who are always at the center. In addition, the center has four mind-counselors and coaches because cancer patients are typically overstressed, and this stress needs to be brought under control.

Counseling helps get rid of stress

When a patient starts the program, one of the counselors asks the patient why they have cancer. Over half of the patients know exactly why they have cancer, but the others have no idea or aren't sure. Lothar believes one of the most important strategies for healing is to get to the root of the problem.

That's why the counselor asks about possible difficulties at work or within the family. A negative situation can create uncontrolled stress that can collapse the immune system, causing cancer to run out of control. So the counselor uses techniques to change the negative past and help the patient make new decisions about traumatic events they've experienced.

Cancer patients are typically so stressed out that their adrenal glands are completely exhausted. Lothar explained, "They have hardly any adrenalin in the body. We focus right away on bringing the stress levels *down*! We do that through such things as meditation, visualization, dancing, singing, and laughing. We explain to the patient why we do all of these things. When the patient is de-stressed, the adrenalin level goes up, which is what we want." For entertainment, patients watch carefully selected movies that contain a lot of comedy to get them laughing.

When patients arrive, a staff member tells them that the center creates a "healing field." If the patient has any kind of problem or difficulty, Lothar insists that they inform the staff right away so any negativity can be cleared up immediately.

Goal setting is another important part of the counseling process. It takes time. Lothar said, "Nobody wants to talk about sexuality, but it's so important. A lot of cancer patients don't have sex with their spouse. But it's important for the patient's energy level. They have to find a way to be happy.

"For one patient out of 10 we never do find out why they have cancer. In those cases we just tell them that if nothing changes, nothing will change. We say, 'You have to change something. This is your life, and your life has brought you to the point when you got cancer. We aren't here to say if your life was good or bad. But if you make no changes whatsoever in your life, what can you expect going forward? More cancer, more metastasis, and death. You must turn either right or left instead of going straight ahead on the same path that produced the cancer.'"

Lothar is astounded that so few cancer doctors pay attention to their patients' adrenalin level. He said, "A doctor in Northern Germany found that if the adrenalin in his patients didn't go up, they all died. You have to bring up the adrenalin level! You can measure this. I can prove this. The adrenalin test is so easy and so helpful. How can you build it up? You can't inject it or give it as an infusion. There's only one way: you have to bring the body's stress level *down*. We want every patient to go to bed with a good, peaceful feeling, and we tell the patients why. Patients must stay on the anti-stress program. The Budwig eating plan and anti-stress are the two most important cancer treatments! Laetrile infusions are fine, but the basics are nutrition, detox, fresh air, and natural sunshine."

Color therapy is another strategy Lothar believes in. Each bathroom has blue lights and red lights. Lothar said, "If people are low in energy, we use blue light when they take their daily bath. If they're too stressed and hopeless, we use red lights."

In addition, rooms are painted different colors. A patient who needs to be "brought down" gets a yellow room. Dark green is for patients who need more energy.

The center also uses music therapy to help deprogram negative thinking and irrational fear.

The importance of detox

Lothar said, "We believe in the self-healing process. This is one of the main things we're doing here. When we help a patient with detox, for example, we love problems. We love it if something happens: diarrhea, insomnia, skin problems, even pain! Why? Because it means the body is starting to repair things. It's okay if the detoxing patient can't sleep a whole night: they don't like it, but it's okay. Nobody likes diarrhea, but the detoxing patient should be happy to be getting rid of unwanted waste.

"The same is true of skin problems: this means poisons are leaving the body through the skin. Some elderly patients think they have bone problems after about two weeks of doing the program because the body is starting to repair the bones. We tell these patients to be happy because in a few days the problem is gone and they feel better and have more energy."

For detox, patients take enemas and baking soda baths every day. Lothar explained that a tumor produces a bad kind of lactate (left spin lactic acid) that must be brought out. He told me, "I don't understand why conventional doctors aren't doing this. Even if they know about it, they don't do anything about it. Lactate is around the tumor, helping the tumor grow. We want to stop this. We want to get the lactate out. Tumors produce lactate 24 hours a day. We have to get it out every day.

"Patients do a baking soda bath by putting 150 grams of baking soda into their hot bathwater. The water must be more than their body temperature, around 101 to 103 degrees Fahrenheit. The pH of the bathwater without the baking soda is around seven. The pH with baking soda goes up to eight. We need it over eight. Lactate has a pH of 6. The patient soaks in the hot baking soda water for 30 minutes, adding hot water every five minutes to keep the water hot.

"After the bath we measure the pH of the bathwater to determine how much lactate came out of the patient's body. *This is a perfect therapy*. It's cheap and easy, which is why no one is interested in it."

Of course, you don't have to go to Germany to start taking baking soda baths. You can start doing it right now in the privacy of your bathroom at home. This daily ritual is also relaxing and de-stressing, which likewise boosts health.

Before the bath, Lothar recommends another low-tech, low-cost effective ritual: dry skin brushing. This ritual renews the skin, stimulates the lymphatic system, boosts circulation, and assists the detox process. You need one brush with a handle for the body, and a finer brush for your face. I personally use the "Skin Brush Combo" from the website BernardJensen.com. This combo costs about $20. Dry skin brushing is a good health habit whether you have cancer or not. Like baking soda baths, it's cheap and easy, which explains why there's little interest in it.

Patients at the center do a coffee enema every day. As you may have heard, coffee enemas detoxify the liver. It plays a key role in the famous Gerson cancer protocol. At Lothar's facility, some patients do two or more of these enemas per day, if necessary. Coffee enemas and baking soda baths also give patients pain relief. Lothar said, "A baking soda bath is sometimes 10 times better than any other pain killer. Get the lactate out, and the pain goes out, too."

In addition, patients get two sessions of colonic hydrotherapy per week. Lothar remarked that nobody wants to do colonic hydrotherapy when they first come to the clinic. But every patient is happy they did it by the end of the five-week program. Each patient also gets at least one liver detox to get rid of stones from the liver and gall bladder.

These machines give patients more energy

In addition to the center's main therapies, certain machines help give the patients more energy. One of these machines is difficult to explain. It exposes the patients to sound waves and light waves, the purpose of which is to change the tension of the cell membrane. The first such machine was built in Switzerland in about 2005. Lothar said, "This machine helps not only cancer patients but others who are low in energy. Some patients do it once or twice a week. Others do it every day."

The center has also gotten spectacular results with another machine that's an electromagnetic device. Prostate patients sit on the business end of the device to get the benefit. Others can put the device wherever the problem area is.

An 18-year-old patient came to the clinic every day for about four weeks – not because she had cancer but because she couldn't hold urine. She sat on the device for a half hour a day. "Now she's fine," said Lothar. "This machine brings electricity to your body. It's unbelievable! You have these machines in America, but the

FDA doesn't allow them to be used as a medical device. Landscapers in America are using them for plants. Yes, it also works for plants. The machine gives energy. That's all it does! A few patients in America are using it under the radar for cancer."

One of the center's most powerful diagnostic tools is a darkfield microscope, which can reveal nasty organisms ("very small animals," as Lothar calls them) in the patient's blood. Lothar said, "After two or three weeks at our center we see fewer animals. In most cases they're gone after five weeks."

"All illnesses are good – at first"

Lothar observed that people assume illness is always bad. On the contrary, Lothar said that illness is always good – at first. Take a fever, for example. A fever is the immune system's attempt to burn out something that's invading the body, and that's good. But you don't want a fever to run out of control because an excessive fever can kill the patient. Another example is diarrhea, which is the body's attempt to get rid of something that's bad. This detox is good, but uncontrolled diarrhea can cause lethal dehydration.

How can a tumor possibly be good? Lothar explained, "A tumor helps to burn down heavy metals in your body. It also collects fungus from your body so it doesn't affect the whole body. A tumor also burns excess sugar in the body. A tumor is just showing the patient there's something wrong in his life, something that's out of balance. The cancer cell is your best friend, at first. Illness is your friend in the beginning."

Patients come for five weeks because that's the shortest time during which they can do the whole program. At least five weeks are needed for the body to repair.

Nine out of 10 patients who enter the five-week program have already given up when they arrive. The center's focus is to give them hope. These patients need to be un-brainwashed and deprogrammed. The center has one German-speaking group of patients, and another English-speaking group. Patients come from the Americas, South Africa, Australia, Russia, and elsewhere. Most of the patients are German. Few French patients come because they generally prefer not to speak English.

Lothar gave me a copy of his book *Chemotherapy Heals Cancer, and the World Is Flat*. He also wrote a book with Budwig about her method. The first half of the book explains her philosophy and eating plan, and the last half contains recipes. This book is the official authorized explanation of how to cure cancer the Budwig way. When I interviewed Lothar, he said the book was available only in German. But by the time you read this, the English translation of *The Great Cookbook and Textbook of the Oil/Protein Diet* may be available.

At the time of this writing, the cost of the the 3E Center's five-week program is 10,300 Euros for all five weeks – only 2,060 per week. This is an astounding bargain. Because it's an in-patient facility, there's no hotel bill on top of the basic charge. A patient's companion can stay at the center for only 840 Euros per week.

If Lothar believes another clinic can better serve a patient, he doesn't hesitate to refer the patient. He knows all of the doctors I interviewed at the various clinics in Germany, Austria, and Switzerland. He has a good relationship with all of them, as the doctors affirmed when I visited them. I'm pleased to see this kind of collegiality and cooperation for the good of the patient.

Contact information:

3E-Zentrum (3E Center)
Im Salenhäule 10
D-73630 Remshalden-Buoch, Germany

Contact: Elke Tegel or Lieselotte Mössner

Website: 3e-Centre.com

e-mail: info@3e-zentrum.de

Phone: 011- 49-7151-9813-201

Fax: 011-49-7151-9813-210

Chapter Four

Dr. Ralf Kleef's Hyperthermia Clinic in Vienna

Dr. Ralf Kleef, M.D., describes himself not as an alternative doctor but as a complementary one. Trained in Germany, Vienna, London, and America, he says the three years he spent doing research at the Memorial Sloan-Kettering Cancer Center in New York followed by one year at the NIH in Washington made him a skeptic. He believes a good scientist should try to prove himself wrong instead of becoming a "true believer" in his own theory.

He told me, "In God we trust. All others must bring data." He's willing to try a therapy that other doctors recommend, but he says, "We throw things out right away if they don't seem to be helpful."

The four years he spent in America also gave him the opportunity to perfect his English, which he speaks with hardly a trace of a German accent.

Before he was accepted for a postdoctoral fellowship at Sloan-Kettering, he was hired at the BioMed Klinik in Bad Bergzabern and worked under that clinic's legendary founder, the late Dieter Hager, M.D. At BioMed he learned about hyperthermia, detoxification, nutrition, and natural medicine.

The best medicine is medicine that *works*!

Dr. Kleef rejects the dichotomy between conventional medicine and natural medicine. Instead, he says there's good medicine and bad medicine. He aims to give his patients the best medicine, whether it's conventional or natural or a combination of both. The best medicine is medicine that *works*.

In 1998 Dr. Kleef founded his own clinic in Vienna, which has become the top hyperthermia center in Austria and one of the leading and most influential hyperthermia centers in all of Europe. His colleagues in Germany and Switzerland attest that he is a leader in his field. He has treated over 8,000 patients, and has had many successes. Like all of the cancer doctors I interviewed in Europe, he also has had some failures when patients came too late.

Patients come from all over the world for treatment by Dr. Kleef. When I visited his clinic he was treating a patient from Australia, a gold miner from Alaska, and others from various parts of the globe. He also has an immunotherapy clinic nearby, which he really wanted to show me. He said, "Patients call it the 'Four Seasons Immunology Clinic.'" We laughed. But because of time constraints I was only able to tour the hyperthermia clinic.

Dr. Kleef told me it's necessary to spend time with each patient. He said, "We ask them, 'Do you want to live? Do you really want to live?' Some are surprised that we ask the question."

Unhappiness, according to Dr. Kleef, is one of the four main causes of cancer. He said, "Many people aren't happy in their lives today. They have no meaning in their lives. This unhappiness, which has become common in society, drives cancer. The first miracle of Jesus was when he turned water into wine at the wedding banquet in Cana. This miracle brought joy to the wedding guests. What people need is joy in their lives."

The three other main causes of cancer are:

- Nutrition. The foods in supermarkets are generally deficient in vitamins and minerals.
- Environmental pollution. Dr. Kleef said, for example, that when women are on "the Pill" (which European doctors call the "anti-baby pill"), they excrete the drug in their urine, and the drug finds its way into the environment.
- Lack of exercise and chronic stress. Dr. Kleef's clinic has a diagnostic machine that assesses the balance of the patient's sympathetic and parasympathetic nervous system. It's crucial for health and healing to bring stress under control.

To control stress, the clinic includes a yoga and meditation room to support the spiritual aspect of healing. The patients are taught meditation and breathing techniques for relaxation.

There are also other causes of cancer. Dr. Kleef believes it's dangerous to have a cell phone glued to your ear, as many young people do. He sees children getting brain cancer, and he believes the cell phone is an obvious culprit. He told me, "If you put an egg between two mobile phones, you'll see the proteins getting cooked." He also remarked that EMF chaos (electromagnetic frequencies), such as wireless local networks may be a factor in disease.

Dr. Kleef's unique approach to hyperthermia and immune therapy

Dr. Kleef has pioneered a unique way of administering moderate whole body hyperthermia that he believes is even more effective than extreme whole body hyperthermia.

Here's the difference: When a German doctor administers extreme whole body hyperthermia, he raises the patient's core body temperature to a plateau of 107 degrees Fahrenheit. This plateau is maintained for about two hours, during which the patient is under anesthesia, carefully monitored, and kept properly hydrated. German doctors have done thousands of these procedures. They know what they're doing. The procedure is safe.

By contrast, Dr. Kleef raises the patient's core body temperature to a moderate fever temperature of 102 degrees Fahrenheit, but he holds it at that plateau for a much longer time: 6 or 7 hours. It takes about three hours to bring the patient's body temperature up to the plateau and another hour for the patient's temperature to come back down to normal. Altogether, Dr. Kleef's unique way of administering moderate whole body hyperthermia can take about 10 hours. He keeps the patient under anesthesia throughout the procedure, during which the patient is closely monitored and kept hydrated.

Dr. Kleef said, "A plateau temperature of 39 degrees Celsius [102 degrees Fahrenheit] is a better immune stimulator than extreme whole body hyperthermia."

In addition to stimulating the immune system, whole body hyperthermia weakens cancer cells so they can be killed by another therapy, such as low-dose chemotherapy.

Chemo sensitivity testing is a must!

But Dr. Kleef condemns the indiscriminate use of chemo because in some cases chemo is ineffective against a patient's cancer. In those cases, chemo would needlessly poison the patient. He believes chemo sensitivity testing is the wave of the future because it tells the doctor which chemotherapy drug, if any, would be effective against an individual patient's strain of cancer cell. If chemo sensitivity testing indicates that a certain chemo drug would be helpful, Dr. Kleef uses a low dose of that drug in combination with hyperthermia and other therapies.

He's proud to say that his clinic also offers hyperthermic intraperitoneal chemo for advanced ovarian, pancreatic, and stomach cancers. As you may know, the peritoneum is the membrane that lines the abdominal cavity and covers most of the abdominal organs. Introducing a heated chemotherapeutic liquid into this cavity is a brilliant way of targeting and killing the cancer cells in the abdomen without harming normal cells. Because cancer cells are sensitive to heat, adding heat to this specialized chemo treatment makes it even more effective.

Dr. Kleef would also like to bring low-dose radiation and whole body hyperthermia under the same roof. While high-dose radiation is toxic, dangerous, and damaging, he believes low-dose radiation can be a useful tool against tough, stubborn cancers. But he cautions not to overuse the diagnostic procedure of PET/CT scans because they give the patient a radiation load that's too heavy. He does infrared thermograms instead, which cause no harm to the patient.

For local hyperthermia, Dr. Kleef uses – parallel to the well-known Oncotherm device – an Italian-made Syncrotherm machine, which he says is more powerful to treat deep-seated lesions than the Oncotherm machines that are used in many other clinics. With each hyperthermia treatment the patient also gets oxygen and ionizing therapy.

Dr. Kleef also offers a specialized form of hyperthermia for prostate cancer patients: transurethral hyperthermia. In this therapy, a catheter with a special heating device is inserted in the urethra through the prostate and into the bladder. Once the catheter is in place, the part with the heating element is positioned inside the prostate. When the heat is turned on, the prostate becomes heated enough to kill the cancer cells without harming the prostate's healthy cells. This remarkable therapy is also an effective treatment for prostatitis and for an enlarged prostate.

Currently, the most promising approach is a combination of immune therapy with hyperthermia: Dr. Kleef oversaw the first cases of Stage Four cancer patients who underwent partial to nearly complete remission by simultaneous low-dose checkpoint inhibitors (LD-IC) in combination with high-dose (HD)-IL-2 treatment and hyperthermia.

He demonstrated the feasibility and safety of this multi-functional treatment approach using immune-based combination therapy without conventional cytotoxic chemotherapy. He says, "Harnessing autoimmune T cells that are activated by a low-dose immune checkpoint blockade could be a safe and powerful tool to defeat late-stage cancer."

Other therapies include:

- Galvano therapy, which gently "zaps" breast cancers and other cancers that are close to the surface of the skin
- Ozone therapy
- Colonic hydrotherapy
- Infusions of high dose vitamin C
- Traditional Chinese medicine: the clinic employs a traditional Chinese medical doctor.

Let me tell you some remarkable stories of patients who came to Dr. Kleef's clinic with difficult, deadly cancers and recovered their health.

Stage Four melanoma patient changed his eating plan

Forty-eight-year-old Andrew M. from Hong Kong was diagnosed with Stage Four malignant melanoma – one of the most difficult cancers of all. His primary tumor was on his cheek, but he also had tumors in his lungs. Dr. Kleef put together a treatment plan that included immune-boosting therapy, long-duration whole body hyperthermia, local hyperthermia, Interleukin 2, checkpoint inhibitors, a vast array of supplements, dietary recommendations, and infusions including vitamin C. As I write this, over one year following his initial diagnosis, he's in complete remission.

Andrew changed his eating plan and lost over 30 unwanted pounds. While he hasn't yet reached the five year survival mark, he says, "I am in good health. I am indebted to Dr. Kleef for his care and attention, his open-mindedness and flexibility, and for his friendship. His whole team has treated me with nothing but love."

Stage Four breast cancer patient almost gave up

Anna W. from the United Kingdom received conventional cancer treatment in London for Grade III triple negative breast cancer. She underwent five grueling months of chemo followed by a lumpectomy, the removal of lymph nodes under her arm, and one month of radiation.

A few months later she was devastated to learn that the cancer had come back. But this time it was worse. It had spread to her lungs. Her London doctor could offer nothing more than palliative care and gave her a death sentence. Her friends started looking for alternative treatments and found my book *German Cancer Breakthrough*. Anna finally decided to go to Vienna for treatment at Dr. Kleef's clinic after consulting with Dr. Ralph Moss.

Her treatment in Vienna, which lasted several weeks, included local and whole body hyperthermia, various infusions, high dose Interleukin 2, and low dose checkpoint inhibitor therapy. She abruptly quit Dr. Kleef's clinic and stopped all treatment because one of the infusions, Taurolidine (an anti-microbial substance), was making her feel awful. It turns out that Anna was intolerant to Taurolidine – the first patient Dr. Kleef has ever had who was!

But when she went back to her London hospital for a checkup, she was amazed to see her chest X-rays: the tumors in her lungs had shrunk. This encouraged her to take the last dose of the checkpoint inhibitor therapy she had brought back from Vienna. A couple of months later, a follow up visit showed that her lung tumors had shrunk even more. So she decided to return to Dr. Kleef's Vienna clinic for another round of Interleukin 2 and the checkpoint inhibitor therapy.

Anna is delighted with the results and even emailed me a series of four X-rays, spaced two months apart, demonstrating the effectiveness of Dr. Kleef's treatment. She highly recommends the clinic and says, "I'm feeling very well and have regained my energy, which is fantastic."

Dr. Kleef spares no effort to help his patients

Although Dr. Kleef is skilled at treating cancer, he strongly prefers that people do what's necessary to prevent it because "prevention is easier than curing Stage Four."

Each patient's treatment is completely individualized: only after lots of testing does Dr. Kleef propose a treatment. He looks at molecular testing, chemo sensitivity testing, the whole microenvironment of the tumor, and other factors to determine the best treatment plan. Dr. Kleef told me, "It's complex, and it takes a lot of work and research."

Dr. Kleef has found that hyperthermia combined with immunotherapy is also effective for a wide range of diseases, including allergies, eczema, inflammatory diseases, autoimmune diseases, chronic pain, Lyme disease, and viral diseases.

Looking out the window from the hyperthermia clinic I could see a huge park. Next to the park is a hotel where Dr. Kleef's outpatients certainly have a pleasant place to stay. For music lovers, Vienna is heaven on earth because of the world-famous Vienna Philharmonic and Vienna State Opera. I'd hoped to attend a concert or an opera, but I only had time to visit the graves of Beethoven, Schubert, and other immortal artists before my appointment with Dr. Kleef.

If you're looking for a first-class cancer clinic and you're a music lover, Dr. Kleef's Vienna clinic is an obvious choice. Even if you're not interested in music, you may want to choose this outstanding clinic in one of the cultural capitals of Europe.

Each cancer case is different, and the cost of treatment depends on what therapies are needed and how long they are necessary. Dr. Kleef's complex new approach of combining immunotherapy (low dose checkpoint inhibitors with high dose IL-2) with hyperthermia would cost around 25,000 to 30,000 Euros for a course of treatment that lasts four to five weeks. This price includes the cost of medication, which is expensive. Patients are provided with an individual cost proposal before they arrive in Vienna.

Contact information:

Dr. Kleef Hyperthermie

Auhofstraße 1-3
A-1130 Vienna, Austria

Contact: Ralf Kleef, M.D.

Website: www.dr-kleef.at/en/

e-mail: office@dr-kleef.at

Phone: 011-43-1585-7311

Fax: 011-43-1585-7311-20

Chapter Five

Dr. Uwe Reuter's Hospital "Klinik im LEBEN" in Greiz

Never before had I been behind the former Iron Curtain. But when I was making arrangements for my third tour of the German cancer clinics I found out about an outstanding clinic in Greiz, a city that was once part of East Germany.

Greiz became a city of opulence when the textile industry was booming in the late 19th and early 20th centuries. In fact, the clinic occupies several of the magnificent century-old buildings from this golden age, built around 1908. Some of the buildings feature stained glass windows, beveled glass, ornately decorated ceilings, elaborate fireplaces, and other forms of craftsmanship rarely found in modern buildings. One of the buildings even contains a private museum of antique medical devices and instruments.

Staying at the clinic as an in-patient is like staying in a palace. Because one of the overnight rooms for patients was vacant, my wife and I spent a night at the clinic. Our room had vintage furniture and also included a balcony overlooking the crystal clear waters of the Weiße Elster river. So clear are the waters that it was easy to see the individual stones at the bottom of the river, even from our third-floor balcony.

Our balcony also overlooked the clinic's Garden of Life – an artistically designed garden with walking paths and a gazebo where patients and staff can relax in nature and meditate.

The hospital "Klinik & Praxis im LEBEN" in Greiz describes itself as an F.X. Mayr house. Dr. F.X. Mayr was an Austrian physician who discovered the elements of a regenerative cure for body, mind, and soul more than 100 years ago. His cure is based on nutrition, digestion, and motion.

The clinic's head physician, Dr. Uwe Reuter, M.D., told me, "Mayr medical treatment begins with fasting and continues with mild food. Our cook is a trained chef for these meals. It's important for us to teach our patients how to eat right with no processed food.

"Digestion takes a lot of energy, depending on what you eat. The food we serve isn't raw because raw food can be hard to digest, especially in the evening. Our eating plan lets the colon rest so it doesn't use a lot of energy in digestion. The colon is important in the treatment."

The clinic combines the theories and practices of Mayr with sophisticated, state-of-the-art technological devices and mild but effective cancer treatments.

Another unique aspect of this clinic is that it's an informal partner with the legendary Paracelsus Klinik in Switzerland. In fact, Dr. Ralf Oettmeier, M.D., a former doctor at the Greiz clinic, is now on the staff at Paracelsus. He's the one who told me about the Greiz clinic and recommended that I visit it.

Greiz does have one advantage over Switzerland: certain therapies that aren't legally permitted in Switzerland are offered in Greiz, such as laetrile therapy and fever therapy with Coley's toxins. When doctors at Paracelsus recognize that a patient needs a therapy that's only offered at the Greiz clinic, the patient is urged to transfer to Greiz. This kind of collegiality and cooperation for the patient's benefit is commendable.

A booklet co-written by Dr. Oettmeier and Dr. Reuter makes an analogy between a computer and the levels of biological systems in a patient. The patient's organs, cells, and biological systems may be compared to a computer's hardware: they're visible and measurable. The patient's flow of energy in the body may be compared to the electric current that flows through a computer: it's invisible but measurable. The patient's psyche, emotions, feelings, beliefs, and intuition are like software: they're invisible and hardly measurable.

Even though the psychological and spiritual aspect of the patient is invisible and difficult to measure, it can have a big impact on health. That's why the clinic considers it so important for patients to replace destructive thoughts with constructive thoughts, to bring stress under control, and to find peace with God.

Several patients at the clinic were eager to tell me their stories.

Conventional treatment would have ruined Regina's life

I interviewed a German lady, Regina, who was at the clinic for followup. Three years ago she came to the Greiz clinic for biological treatment of her tongue cancer after refusing conventional radiation treatments that would have destroyed her salivary glands. Not being able to produce saliva would have ruined her quality of life.

Her daughter told her about Greiz. Regina told me, speaking through an interpreter, that she got a good welcome at Greiz and that every treatment is well explained so she knows exactly what will happen. She likes that.

Like all patients, when she first came to the clinic she went through a battery of diagnostic tests, including darkfield microscopy, a blood test, a saliva test, thermography, electronic acupuncture, and a stress test to assess the balance between the sympathetic and parasympathetic nervous system. Stress control is crucial for cancer patients because uncontrolled stress weakens the immune system.

When the diagnostics were complete, the doctors put together a treatment plan for Regina, which included local hyperthermia for her tongue, whole body hyperthermia, and fever therapy with Coley's toxins (a special house mixture). Dr. Reuter said the hyperthermia and fever treatment were crucial to her recovery. Regina remarked that she especially liked the local hyperthermia and fever therapy. The fever therapy caused her to shiver a bit, but after an hour she was okay.

During whole body hyperthermia, the doctors brought her body temperature up to 39 to 40 degrees Celsius (102 to 104 degrees Fahrenheit) and held it in that range for at least three hours. For some patients, doctors bring the body temperature a little higher – up to 40 to 41 degrees Celsius (104 to 106 degrees celsius). The German doctors have vast experience with hyperthermia and know how to do it safely.

Regina's active fever therapy with Coley's toxins started in the morning, and it caused a fever that lasted about six to eight hours. Three days are needed for fever therapy. Day one is for preparation. Day two is for administering the therapy. Day three is detox day to get rid of the dead tumor tissue. Fever therapy can't be given more than twice a week. Usually, fever therapy is alternated with whole body hyperthermia. Patients can get local hyperthermia every day.

Before Regina knew about the Greiz clinic, she had had one surgery to remove tonsils and lymph nodes. She wishes that she had come to the Greiz clinic before having that surgery because she believes it was unnecessary. She never did have any kind of surgery on her cancerous tongue, which healed up completely as a result of the biological treatment in Greiz.

Detox foot baths and colonic hydrotherapy were also a part of Regina's treatment plan. In addition, she did physical therapy, received infusions with curcumin and other substances, and took homeopathic remedies.

Regina loves the clinic. She has told all of her friends and neighbors about how she got rid of her tongue cancer without surgery and without the ruinous effects of radiation. They can hardly believe she looks so good.

Frank was given two or three days to live

I interviewed a German named Frank, who also spoke to me through an interpreter. Four years earlier doctors had discovered he had a dangerous tumor next to his aorta and heart. The tumor was so large it was inoperable. His conventional doctors could only offer chemo, which he realized was no permanent solution. So he refused.

Two years ago he heard about the Greiz clinic and started receiving treatment with biological medicine there, but he still had trouble getting his stress under control. In fact, his stress was so bad that it cancelled out the benefits of his biological treatments. A few months later he had a health crisis, and he was taken to the hospital by ambulance.

He was told he had two or three days to live – a week at most. That put the fear of God into him! He immediately decided to take responsibility for himself and for his healing. The Greiz clinic helped him get his stress under control through meditation and mind-body medicine. He also found spiritual peace.

Dr. Reuter said that Frank had 22 fever therapies plus local and whole body hyperthermia. Frank firmly believes that the Greiz clinic is "the best possible way." He said, "There should be more clinics like this." He's certain that he owes his life to this clinic.

Conventional doctor Stephanie: "You need ch else you'll die"

Stephanie is a 47-year-old German woman who works in the insurance industry. When I interviewed her, she told me it's important for her to say that she *had* breast cancer – past tense. She's proud to say she's cancer free, and she readily gives credit to the Greiz clinic. She was at the clinic for followup treatments, including local hyperthermia, to keep the cancer from sneaking back. She told me she feels perfectly healthy, and her blood results and tumor markers are excellent.

She especially loves the local hyperthermia treatments, during which she lies down on a water bed and never fails to fall asleep.

Five years earlier she was diagnosed with an aggressive form of breast cancer on her left side. Her only conventional treatment was a minor operation (lumpectomy) that left her breast intact. Her conventional doctors told her, "You need chemo, or else you'll die!" But she didn't trust them. Her mother took chemotherapy, which made her feel rotten and killed her. So Stephanie refused chemo and radiation. When her cancer came back, she had another lumpectomy. Again, she resisted the bullying of doctors who tried to push her into chemo and radiation.

About a year ago she found out about the Greiz clinic and started treatment there. In addition to local hyperthermia, she had infusions and various dietary supplements, including vitamins, minerals, enzymes, and selenium. She loves these treatments because they are gentle but effective, allowing her to maintain an excellent quality of life with none of the misery associated with chemotherapy and radiation. She can't recommend the clinic highly enough.

The clinic's website describes other successful case studies.

The clinic's Garden of Life for patients and staff

The gate leading to the clinic's Garden of Life, which is right next to the river, is a symbol of division between the stresses and pressures of daily life and another world – a world of peace and tranquility. This private garden is open to patients, their companions, and clinic staff.

The paths through the garden include a bridge over running water. There are goldfish in the pond. Every place in the garden has a symbolic meaning, as indicated by various signs. For example, stones signify the difficulties in life. The clinic encourages patients to consider a trip through the garden as a way to make a symbolic journey and to peacefully contemplate how to get better and how to proceed in life.

The garden includes a vegetable patch. Gardening tools are available for patients who enjoy gardening, which is considered one of the best forms of exercise. Various structures, such as a gazebo and pergola, give patients several places to sit down, slow down, and contemplate, meditate, or pray in a peaceful, beautiful, tranquil setting.

Transurethral hyperthermia and other specialized treatments

During my tour of the clinic, the staff showed me a wide array of treatments available. One of the most remarkable treatments, which is highly effective for prostate cancer that hasn't spread beyond the prostate, is transurethral hyperthermia. Each treatment requires an unusual catheter that passes through the prostate into the bladder.

What's unusual about the catheter is that it contains a specialized heating element that heats up the prostate from inside. This heat kills or damages the cancer cells without harming the prostate's normal cells.

The clinic has found that three transurethral hyperthermia treatments over a three-week period are usually enough to knock out the prostate cancer without damaging the prostate.

Transurethral hyperthermia is inexpensive. Each treatment costs only 925 Euros. It's worth mentioning that this treatment can also be effective for treating benign prostate hyperplasia (BPH), also known as an "enlarged prostate" – a common problem in older men. Many prostate cancer patients also have BPH.

One of the best treatments for breast cancer and other cancerous areas (except the bones and brain) is Galvano therapy. Electrodes are connected to the affected area, and a low voltage current (35 volts) is applied. This therapy wakes up hydrochloric acid, which destroys the membrane behind which cancer cells hide, while leaving normal cells undamaged. Afterward, the patient is given injections for detox to get rid of the dead cancer cells.

Because cancer cells hate oxygen, the clinic uses oxygen and ozone therapies. Other therapies include:

- Magnetic field therapy to boost the immune system and increase microcirculation of the blood
- Ozone therapy
- Ultraviolet blood irradiation
- Massage therapy, including hot stone massage
- Ayurvedic medicine and traditional Chinese medicine

No toxic chemicals, no electro-magnetic frequency chaos

The clinic is serious about providing patients with a safe environment that's as free as possible from toxins and electro-magnetic frequency (EMF) chaos.

The furniture is made from natural materials only, and it's not treated with chemicals or any toxic substances. The flooring, too, is made of natural substances only, such as cork, which is also an excellent insulator. There is no PVC (polyvinyl chloride) in any of the buildings. To spare patients from exposure to negativity and bad news, there are no televisions in the patients' rooms. But if a patient requests a TV, the clinic will provide one.

What patients can expect

Each patient gets an individualized treatment plan after going through a thorough series of diagnostic tests. The basic treatment typically lasts two or three weeks, depending on how severe the cancer is. When the treatment is completed, the clinic gives the patient homework – what they should do and shouldn't do when they go home. They also get instructions on how to keep up the F.X. Myer eating plan. In addition, they get pharmaceutical-grade vitamins, minerals, and supplements to support their health.

The cost is surprisingly reasonable, considering the elegant, beautifully preserved historic facilities. The basic weekly rate for patients is 5,572 Euros, which includes room, board, diagnostic tests, deep local hyperthermia, moderate whole-body hyperthermia, most other therapies, and shuttle service to and from each German airport (for patients staying two weeks or more).

Medicines and special treatments are extra. For example, each treatment of transurethral hyperthermia costs 925 Euros. Three such treatments are usually given in a three week period – one per week.

In-patients are encouraged to stay with a companion, who is charged only 520 Euros per week for room and board. To be picked up at the airport, patients may fly into Berlin, Munich, or Frankfurt. The closest major cities are Leipzig and Dresden.

Outpatients have a choice of several options for lodging, including the highly-rated Bio-See Hotel and Spa in Zeulenroda, which is located right next to an enormous lake. At sunset I enjoyed a fine dinner in the restaurant at the top floor of this hotel, and the view was spectacular. This hotel is popular with outpatients who come to the clinic from China and elsewhere. The clinic can give advice for other lodging options.

The clinic's website features a short video tour. In addition to treating cancer, the clinic also provides effective holistic treatment for other chronic conditions including autoimmune diseases, Lyme disease, and pain.

Contact information:

Hospital "Klinik im LEBEN"

Gartenweg 5-6
D-07973 Greiz, Germany

Contact: Ines Schubert

Website: klinik-imleben.de

e-mail: kontakt@klinik-imleben.de

Phone: 011-49-3661-6898-70

Fax: 011-49-3661-6898-72

Chapter Six

Dr. Andreas Demuth's Hufeland Klinik in Bad Mergentheim

"There's some kind of energy in this place that's extremely healing," raved one satisfied patient

The world-famous Hufeland Klinik is located in the charming city of Bad Mergentheim, which is known for its historic cityscape, the healing waters of its naturally mineralized springs, and its enchanting views of the surrounding countryside.

The first thing that hits you when you walk into the 55-bed Hufeland Klinik is that it doesn't look or smell at all like a hospital. Rather, the atmosphere is warm and welcoming.

The head of the Hufeland Klinik is Dr. Andreas M. Demuth, M.D. (pronounced Daymoot). He's a brilliant, young, mild-mannered physician who speaks English flawlessly.

In a typical month, the clinic treats two American patients. Patients have come from at least 34 countries all over the world. And unlike some clinics, Hufeland accepts children as patients.

Right off the bat, I asked Dr. Demuth to tell me about some tough cases in which he had really "turned cancer around." He did tell me about amazing histories, as you'll discover for yourself in a moment.

A different approach to both disease and healing

But Dr. Demuth said if you look to a doctor to "turn cancer around," you're looking at the problem as conventional medicine does. "Healing can't be forced," he said.

Dr. Demuth emphasized that it's really the *patient* who turns his own cancer around because healing is a mysterious power that comes from *within* the patient. The Hufeland Klinik offers some of the most effective therapies known to man, but the patient must awaken his or her inner healing powers so the therapies will really kick in and kick the cancer out.

Instead of presenting himself as the "boss" who "leads" the patient to health, Dr. Demuth sees himself as the patient's guide and companion, walking side-by-side with the patient toward better health. This approach is the polar opposite of what American patients are used to. But the American patient I interviewed really liked the clinic and recommended it to other Americans without reservation.

To turn cancer around, Dr. Demuth says you must engage the patient's psychological, mental, and spiritual resources. And that's why his clinic applies the breakthrough counseling techniques of the late American pioneer O. Carl Simonton, M.D. Ironically, some of Germany's finest doctors are using Dr. Simonton's life-saving techniques, while most American doctors largely ignore them.

In fact, shortly before Dr. Simonton's death, I interviewed him by phone from his home. I included a chapter about him in my book *America's Best Cancer Doctors and Their Secrets*. You can get more information about this book from the CancerDefeated.com website. Just click on the link "Publications."

By the time many patients discover Hufeland, their doctor has already told them they have "three months" or "six months" to live. Yet no doctor can possibly know how much time a patient has. Through counseling, the clinic seeks to unbrainwash and deprogram the patients from these predictions.

Dr. Demuth told me, "The second diagnosis is the worst. When the patient is first diagnosed with cancer, the patient may be optimistic that the cancer can be fixed with chemo and radiation. But when the cancer comes back after chemo and radiation, a deep shock sets in, and the patients ask, 'How could this happen?' They're physically weakened and psychologically devastated. Yet they can be encouraged that it's still possible to pull out of it."

According to Dr. Demuth, people set themselves up for cancer by tolerating a lot of stress in their lives and eating a poor diet. Conversely, the way to get rid of cancer is to reduce stress by learning how to manage it, and to eat nutritious organic food along with effective nutritional supplements. The Hufeland Klinik makes sure each patient is educated about nutrition and stress management.

I also interviewed Dr. Gerhard Balthasar, who specializes in homeopathy, general medicine, fever therapy, and acupuncture. Dr. Balthasar was eager to talk to me. He's fluent in English, French, Dutch, Italian, and, of course, his native German.

I asked Dr. Balthasar, "So you don't believe in the cut-burn-poison approach to treating cancer?" He replied, "It's not a question of believing. It's a question of what works best."

How counseling awakens the patient's inner healing forces

Dr. Demuth says if cancer is the problem, patients must be helped to realize that they have more resources at their disposal than "the problem" has. The patient must see that his own resources outweigh the problem.

The medical pioneer who founded the Hufeland Klinik in 1985 was Dr. Wolfgang Woeppel. This is how he expressed his view of cancer:

"The tumor is only the late-stage symptom of cancer, which is from the beginning a systemic disease caused by the impaired working of the body's own defense and repair mechanisms. Cancer is not merely the disorder of one organ but is an expression of a comprehensive disorder of the whole person in his or her unity of body and soul. Traditional European naturopathy, empirical medicine, and conventional scientific medicine can be selectively used in a unique way that rebuilds people instead of destroying them."

Today, the clinic is run by Dr. Woeppel's widow, Frau Gabriele Woeppel, and their lovely daughter Angelika. They are dedicated to maintaining the vision and high standards of the clinic's legendary founder.

Columbia University researchers are impressed with Hufeland cancer success stories

American cancer researchers generally frown on alternative, complementary, and integrative treatments for cancer. But researchers from Columbia University in New York examined several success stories from Hufeland and admitted that "Hufeland treatment merits further study."

This study was published in *Integrative Cancer Therapies*, Vol. 4, No. 2, 2005, pages 156-167. The study also appears online on Hufeland's website: www.hufeland.com. Click on the British flag for the English-language website.

The "healing energy" in Bad Mergentheim

Here's how one patient described the healing energy of Bad Mergentheim:

"You know, there's something about this town. I don't know if you've noticed it. I don't know what it is. But I felt it immediately here. I always feel good when I'm here. Always. There's a good sort of healing energy. That's a good way to describe it. You should go out in that spa park across the street. There's some kind of energy in this place that's extremely healing.

"There are three different springs in the park. Each one has a different name. One of them is the Wilhelm Spring. I combine water from two of the springs. You can buy a cup for 25 cents or else bring your own cup and get the mineralized spring water for free. Every day I go in to get my water and drink it."

The healing waters of the Bad Mergentheim springs

Hufeland doesn't have to persuade the patients to go to the spa park across the street. They go there on their own. Some of them go dancing in the park during the outdoor concerts. And just about all of them avail themselves of the healing waters of the *quelle*, which means "spring" in German.

Spa towns feature naturally mineralized waters that people who seek healing can soak in or drink. The water in each *quelle* boasts its own unique mineral composition.

According to Hufeland's doctors, it's more beneficial to drink the spring water than to soak in it because drinking it gives patients the full benefit of the minerals. One doctor told me that the Wilhelmquelle "is particularly beneficial for the bowels. If you have a glass of Wilhelm's every morning, no bowels can resist it."

In other words, don't drink from the Wilhelmquelle unless you have ready access to a restroom. I would have sampled the water from Wilhelm's spring except that I had to get to my next destination. The water from the heavily mineralized Wilhelmquelle has an off-taste, but Hufeland's patients find the health benefits well worth it.

Hufeland promotes the health discoveries of the legendary 19th century German priest, Fr. Sebastian Kneipp, who cured himself of "incurable" tuberculosis through water therapy alone. The spa park across the street from the clinic has a shallow Kneipp pool that anybody can use to get a refreshing foot bath to improve the circulation of the blood.

The ingenious therapy that had a devastating effect on Barbara's metastasized breast cancer

A lady named Barbara from Northern Germany had a lumpectomy for her breast cancer. She received chemotherapy until 1998. When cancer reappeared in her other breast she underwent another lumpectomy. By December, 2005, her cancer had metastasized.

In March, 2006, she went to the Hufeland Klinik for treatment. Dr. Demuth helped her attack the cancer from several angles.

One of the most effective therapies in her case was Insulin Potentiation Therapy (IPT), which defeated Barbara's cancer with virtually no side effects.

Here's how IPT works: Cancer cells can hide from the immune system, and they're sometimes unaffected by chemotherapy drugs. But they *love* sugar. They need it. They crave it. They thrive on it.

Step One in IPT is to starve the cancer cells of sugar by lowering the patient's blood sugar level. Dr. Demuth achieves this with insulin.

Step Two takes place when the cancer cells are *really* hungry for some sugar. Dr. Demuth gives the cancer cells some sugar, along with a *low* dose of chemo. This clever technique "tricks" the cancer cells into letting their guard down. They eagerly slurp up the sugar right along with the chemo.

The result of IPT is that the *cancer cells* get poisoned, *not* the patient, thanks to the low dose. This is vastly different from the typical American high-dose approach to chemo, which sometimes poisons cancer cells and always poisons the patient.

Barbara had received two cycles of IPT treatments along with antioxidant and enzyme therapy and other therapies. Her treatment was successful.

How Helmut's attitude helped him whip stage four colon cancer with metastasis to the liver

One of the Hufeland patients accepted for the Columbia University study is Helmut, a German who was born in 1943. In June, 1994, he was diagnosed with colon cancer that had metastasized to the liver. His liver cancer was inoperable. This kind of cancer is a virtual death sentence in America. Doctors cut out half of his colon, but they couldn't remove the cancer cells that had spread to his liver.

Helmut had "Stage 4" cancer. In other words, he was at the end of his rope. From 1994 to 1995 he had suffered through nine cycles of 5FU, perhaps the most poisonous chemotherapy drug known. A nickname for 5FU is "five feet under."

As a last resort, Helmut sought treatment at Hufeland and was admitted in May, 1995. By September, his liver metastases were completely gone. He remained in complete remission at the time I wrote this. To say this is remarkable would be an understatement.

Dr. Demuth attributes this success not just to the treatments at the Hufeland Klinik but also to Helmut's psychological attitude. The patient's attitude is of paramount importance: the right attitude leads toward healing, and the wrong attitude leads toward death.

Surprisingly, Helmut accepted the possibility that his cancer could cause his death. Helmut examined his life and said, "Well, maybe I'll make it to the age of 52 in a couple of months. My family is okay. My house is paid for. If I die from this cancer, things will be okay. If my life is over, it's over."

Your common sense might tell you that's the wrong attitude. You might think cancer patients should deny the possibility of death and struggle and fight against it. Not so!

In other words, it would be a mistake for a patient to say, "I'll never accept this cancer! I'll fight the cancer in every way no matter what, etc." That's the wrong attitude.

Dr. Demuth is convinced that Helmut's serene acceptance of the *possibility* that the cancer could kill him was exactly the right attitude. That's because this attitude of *acceptance* enabled Helmut to relax enough to assess his inner resources and focus on health and healing.

My interview with long-term survivor Helmut

Helmut doesn't speak English, but I was able to interview him at Hufeland through an interpreter while he was there for a followup visit. He was a porcelain painter, and he may have gotten his cancer from the toxic substances in his work environment. His cancer seemed just about hopeless. Yet he got rid of it at Hufeland and has remained cancer free.

I asked Helmut, "What's your secret for keeping cancer from coming back?" He replied that he returns to the clinic once a year for intensive immuno-biological therapy. At home, he continues the therapy in cooperation with his family doctor. He follows the recommended eating plan. He doesn't eat a lot of meat. He eats lots of fruits and vegetables and avoids refined sugar. And he exercises faithfully. He's still active as a soccer player, and he enjoys riding a bicycle around Bad Mergentheim. (Hufeland provides bicycles for the patients.)

I asked him, "How is the treatment at Hufeland?" He replied that it isn't painful or stressful. He had absolutely no energy when he first came to the clinic, and he said his quality of life is a lot better when he follows the program. "It's not a miracle. You can support the healing processes in the body," he said.

Helmut said he only tried the Wilhelmquelle one time, and that was it! Apparently, he couldn't tolerate the terrible taste. When I visited the spa park, I wanted to fill my water bottle with water from the Wilhelmquelle to drink it at a later time, but the building in which the spring is located wasn't yet open.

Although Helmut's attitude of acceptance helped him overcome his cancer, some patients carry this attitude *too* far. For example, Dr. Demuth says that some patients tell him, "I'm grateful for my cancer because so many things have changed and I've learned a lot about myself and my loved ones and my attitude toward things." Dr. Demuth instructs the patient to *stop* being grateful for the cancer because the goal is to get rid of it.

Be careful what you focus on, says Dr. Demuth, because what you focus on tends to grow. If you focus all of your attention on cancer, you're likely to get more stress and more cancer. If you focus instead on health and healing, you're likely to get more health and healing.

Viola's story of recovery from breast cancer

In 1996 a German lady named Viola, who was born in 1951, got breast cancer on her left side. It was an aggressive, nasty tumor. Conventional doctors gave her three cycles of chemo, which seemed to solve the problem. But the cancer came back ten years later.

When Viola came to Hufeland, her tumor was large, ugly, and smelly. She was in a great deal of pain, but surgery wasn't possible. During her four weeks of treatment at Hufeland she got immuno-biological therapy in combination with low-dose chemo. I saw "before" and "after" photographs showing her dramatic improvement after the four weeks of therapy.

She improved enough to have surgery after that, and she has been in complete remission ever since then.

The dreadful damage of traditional cancer treatments

Because Dr. Demuth usually sees cancer patients after they've gone through conventional treatments, he's well aware of the harsh effects.

The main side effect of surgery is scar tissue, which can sometimes cause problems. Dr. Demuth said the side effects from the narcotics used to control pain after surgery can last for a year or more. He added that high-dose chemotherapy damages the body and diminishes healing resources for 18 months to two years. But the body can recover from the effects of chemotherapy with good nutritional support.

But Dr. Demuth warned, "After conventional radiation treatment, the body can never recover. You always have side effects, but not visible side effects. The patient can't *feel* the radiation, so conventional doctors cavalierly say, 'Radiation treatment was tolerated very well by the patient.' But what about later? The white blood cell count goes down *for life*! Not much can be done to undo that damage."

Manfred *should* have died from his inoperable metastasized kidney cancer

Manfred, a 62-year-old German, was diagnosed with right-side kidney cancer in November, 2003. Alarmingly, 14 months later an MRI showed that his cancer had metastasized widely. It was inoperable.

In desperation, his doctors started him on the harsh, toxic chemo drug 5FU. But the cancer spread even farther, invading the liver and other organs. Because the chemo wasn't working, he stopped taking it.

As a last resort, Manfred came to Hufeland in July, 2005, for alternative and complementary therapies. By November, 2005, he was in partial remission. By April, 2006, he was in complete remission, as an MRI scan confirmed.

A year later Manfred, who *should* have been long since dead according to the expectations of his conventional doctors, went back to Hufeland for a follow-up visit. He continues to do well.

The gravely ill businessman who *couldn't* die before finishing his task!

A gravely ill insurance executive came to Dr. Demuth in desperation, explaining that he *couldn't* die because he hadn't yet finished his task.

The man's health situation was *beyond bad*. His skin was pure yellow. Dr. Demuth tested his liver function, which was zero! Even Dr. Demuth didn't think he could keep him going for more than a couple of weeks.

The man explained, "I need to pass on the knowledge of how to run my family business to my daughter, and that's going to take six months. I've *got* to keep going for six months. Can you help me?"

Dr. Demuth didn't want to throw a wet blanket on the man's goal to live six months, so he honestly said, "I don't know. But let's try. Let's begin some therapies, and see what we can accomplish working together."

The patient had such a strong mental attitude about the need to keep going for the sake of his family that he was able to complete his task. His heart was full of love for his family, and that was his motivation. This abiding love brought much healing energy into his life.

He met his goal of passing on to his daughter all the knowledge she needed to run the family business. Then, shortly after the six-month grace period, he died in peace at home with his family, surrounded by their love.

Should this case be counted as a failure because the man died of his disease? Some

would say yes. But Dr. Demuth considers it a success because he helped the man reach his goal. No one can deny that the man had a peaceful death.

Dr. Demuth declares, "If we see death as a fault or a failure, then no doctor can be successful. Everybody has to die sometime."

Children get rid of brain cancer at Hufeland

Some of Hufeland's most impressive successes are with brain cancer, which conventional doctors usually consider a death sentence. Dr. Demuth told me about three young boys he treated for brain cancer.

One of these boys was just a year old. His parents brought him to Hufeland after other doctors had given him conventional treatment. Dr. Demuth said he has been stable since 2002, according to a CAT scan.

Today all three of these young former brain cancer patients are healthy. Conventional doctors have a tendency to think "that's impossible" or "it's luck," or "it's a mistake." But no one can deny that these three boys had brain cancer. The proof is undeniable. And so is the proof of their recovery.

One of my personal friends is the father of a child who beat cancer with the help of the Hufeland clinic. My friend is from England, and his name is Kevin Wright. His son's recovery from neuroblastoma, one of the deadliest cancers that strikes children, is so extraordinary that the Cancer Control Society invited him to give a speech at its 2007 annual convention in Universal City, California.

Kevin believes the Hufeland Klinik is a top-notch cancer clinic for children. And his struggle to save his son's life has made him perhaps the most passionate and effective advocate in the world for children who have cancer.

Conventional doctors don't grasp what cancer truly is

Dr. Demuth says cancer is "never, ever, ever a local problem." In other words, doctors shouldn't fall for the trap of thinking that breast cancer is confined to the breast, or prostate cancer is confined to the prostate.

Rather, Dr. Demuth says, "Cancer is a systemic disease involving the mind, the body, the soul, and the spirit. Patients sometimes ask me, 'Do you think whole body hyperthermia is the most important aspect in my treatment plan?' I reply that there are four wheels on a bus. Is the right front wheel the most important one? That makes no sense. Each of us is a body, mind, soul, and spirit. We need these four wheels."

Conventional cancer treatment is so often unsuccessful because it fails to take into account the systemic nature of the disease. Doctors can cut, burn, or poison cancer out of a prostate or breast, but the cancer tends to sneak back. To get rid of the disease for good, you have to address the cause and heal the whole person, including the psychological and spiritual aspects of the patient.

Dr. Demuth offers this advice to anyone with cancer: biopsy and surgery go together. If you're not going to have surgery, you shouldn't have a biopsy. That's because biopsies can spread cancer cells. He also says if you don't want more chemo, you don't need a CAT scan.

He says, "I don't treat cancer, you see, in terms of the tumor. I try to change the milieu in which the cancer is growing. The tumor is only the *expression* of the disease, and the disease is much more complex. So I try to improve the environment in the body. When you change the surroundings, the tumor shrinks."

I asked Dr. Demuth: "So you're saying that changing the environment is what makes cancer shrink, like turning on a light switch and watching the cockroaches run away?" He agreed with that analogy.

Amazingly effective procedures and treatments at the Hufeland Klinik

The treatment program at the Hufeland's 40-bed in-patient clinic begins with detoxification. Indeed, the clinic focuses like a laser beam on detox during the first three weeks of treatment.

To detox the colon, Hufeland patients undergo colonic hydrotherapy. The colon of the typical American or European is a toxic mess from eating too much processed food and junk food and not enough fiber. And when the colon is a toxic mess, the entire body gets poisoned to some degree.

For a cancer patient, job one is to clean the colon. There's no faster or more effective way to flush toxins out of the colon than colonic hydrotherapy. It's mind boggling that something so obvious and important as this is ignored in practically all American cancer hospitals.

In addition, the clinic uses a form of water therapy known as the "permanent shower." The patient takes this warm shower in a horizontal position while the shower device goes back and forth horizontally for an hour and a half. I had never heard of this, and I don't know of any other clinic that has it. This therapy helps the patient detoxify through the skin.

Vaccinations add to the toxic load

While discussing toxicity with Dr. Demuth, he mentioned that he has long believed that vaccinations are an unnecessary source of toxicity. He said that over-vaccination in childhood is a serious problem.

Dr. Demuth has three sons. His first son was vaccinated during his first three years, and then Dr. Demuth decided to stop vaccinating him. His other two boys are completely unvaccinated. His oldest son has an abnormal immune system as a result of the childhood vaccinations: he doesn't get a fever when he gets sick, just a terrible cough for weeks. By contrast, Dr. Demuth's youngest son gets a high fever for two or three days when he gets sick, and then he snaps out of it "better than new."

The importance of a healthy eating plan

A healthy diet also helps move toxins *out* of the body, whereas an unhealthful diet *adds* to the body's toxic load. The Hufeland eating plan emphasizes vegetables and fruits. The grains in the diet are *whole* grains.

The Hufeland strategy is to *alkalize* the body because an alkaline environment is unfriendly to cancer cells. Cancer loves an acidic body. The right nutrition – a diet that emphasizes fruits and vegetables – helps to alkalize the body.

Dr. Demuth says it makes no sense at all for patients to be vegetarian at Hufeland for three weeks and then to go back to their old eating habits. He says a *permanent* lifestyle change is needed. The patient shouldn't go on a "*diet*" but should follow a healthful and flavorful eating plan for life.

The clinic's cafeteria serves quark, which is quite similar to cottage cheese. I was pleased that the clinic recommends a mixture of quark and flax oil, which is the Budwig protocol for cancer treatment. The Budwig diet is perhaps the most effective anti-cancer diet known to man. Americans who want to follow the Budwig protocol can use cottage cheese as a substitute for quark.

Sugar is *verboten*

Refined sugar is *verboten* at the clinic. Refined sugar feeds cancer. Eating lots of fresh, organic vegetables is strongly recommended.

Hufeland's dining room is a pleasant place indeed. Looking out the window you can see the impressive twin towers of a historic church – the *Schloss Kirche*, which means the "castle church."

To further support nutrition, Hufeland patients undergo infusions of intravenous antioxidant therapy with vitamin C, selenium, B-complex and homoepathics. The antioxidants quench the free radicals that would otherwise run loose in the body, causing it to break down.

The spacious area where patients get their IV therapy includes floor-to-ceiling mirrors so that every patient gets a window view, even if their seat faces a wall. One of the windows overlooks the picturesque *Schwarzwald Haus* (Black Forest House).

Because cancer hates oxygen, an essential part of the Hufeland program is supplemental oxygen therapy as well as ozone therapy.

Patients at Hufeland take enzyme therapy to relieve inflammation. The Germans, who pioneered enzyme therapy, have discovered that enzymes eat away the acid wall behind which cancer cells hide from the immune system. This permits the immune system cells to identify and kill the cancer cells.

German doctors use an *American* discovery to defeat cancer!

One of Dr. Demuth's most effective treatments is the "fever push."

Ironically, it was an American doctor, Peter Busch, M.D., who in 1868 discovered by accident that fever can cure cancer. One of his patients was a 43-year-old woman with a severe case of sarcoma of the face. He observed that her cancer went away after she suffered a 105 degree Fahrenheit fever from a strep infection. A fever – whether caused by an illness or artificially induced – has a devastating effect on some forms of cancer.

Yet few American doctors today even know about this remarkable treatment that causes no side effects!

Why does fever therapy work? It's simple: cancer doesn't tolerate heat very well. Fever therapy has a direct effect on cancer cells, killing or weakening them.

Fortunately this bit of medical wisdom hasn't been forgotten. As I've said in previous chapters, German clinics typically use fever therapy (in which the fever is induced by an injection) or hyperthermia (in which the body's temperature is raised by an artificial device) or both.

Dr. Demuth uses *both* methods of raising the patient's body temperature.

In the first kind, he induces a fever reaction by giving the patient mistletoe or interferon A. For a brief time, this causes the patient to feel as if he has an infection. After two hours the patient shivers and feels achy. But because it's not a *real* infection, the fever and its symptoms vanish after a few hours, having severely damaged the cancer cells.

Dr. Demuth has vast experience with this therapy, which is administered to a patient once a week. He's a big fan of mistletoe extract, which stimulates and boosts the immune system. He says it has no downside.

The second kind of therapy that raises the body's temperature is called hyperthermia, which I've described earlier.

The terminology – "fever therapy" and "hyperthermia" – can be a little confusing. When Dr. Demuth talks about "fever therapy," which he also calls a "fever push," he specifically refers to the method of inducing the fever with an injection. He says hyperthermia is a *different* therapy, though it also raises the patient's body temperature.

But some other clinics use "fever therapy" to mean hyperthermia only.

Available *only* in Germany

In Germany, local hyperthermia is done with radio frequencies (short waves), which penetrate deep into the body – 18 centimeters, which is nearly seven inches. This kind of hyperthermia is available only in Germany, Austria, and Switzerland.

Clinics in some countries offer local hyperthermia using microwaves, which only penetrate the body about five centimeters

– approximately two inches. This is far less effective than the deeper penetrating radio frequencies that German doctors use. Hyperthermia with radio frequency waves is not yet available in the United States. Indeed, *any* kind of hyperthermia is difficult to find in America, although acceptance is growing, especially for local (as opposed to whole-body) hyperthermia.

The miracle from space-age technology: Magnetic-field therapy

Hufeland, like almost all of the other German clinics I visited, uses magnetic-field therapy as an important part of the treatment plan. This therapy, which was actually discovered by space scientists for the benefit of astronauts, is much simpler to use than whole-body hyperthermia. It can take place *every* day. The patient simply lies down on a special kind of mat, and when the switch is turned on, a strong magnetic field surrounds the patient while the patient relaxes.

Magnetic-field therapy lasts less than an hour, and it gives patients many benefits: It promotes circulation, boosts the oxygenation of cells, and stimulates energy. Dr. Demuth said that studies prove it promotes bone growth, too. He told us that people today have a deficit in terms of the natural magnetic field because of all the electromagnetic chaos in our modern society. And he says magnetic-field therapy is the solution.

Because magnetic-field therapy promotes circulation and oxygenation, patients have reported improvement with a variety of conditions, including:

- Arthritis
- High blood pressure
- Diabetes
- Stress
- Thyroid conditions
- Skin problems
- Asthma

- Ulcers
- A.D.H.D.
- M.S.
- Cancer

Patients find magnetic-field therapy soothing and relaxing, and they look forward to it every day.

The cornerstone of Hufeland's counseling program is art therapy. Patients paint with watercolors or model with clay. Even patients with no artistic background discover hidden artistic talents. They enjoy creating the artworks and discussing them with the counselor.

Art therapy relaxes the patients and helps them open up to the counselor. In turn, the counselor helps them re-frame their thinking. The counselor helps them see that their inner resources are stronger than cancer.

Patients at Hufeland also enjoy "light therapy" plus music therapy. In a private room, the patient chooses a color and sits in a vibrating massage chair while being bathed in the light of that color and listening to music. Light therapy isn't one of the main therapies at Hufeland, but patients find it relaxing and enjoyable.

Patients tap into spiritual power in Hufeland's chapel

Besides psychological counseling using the Simonton method, patients are encouraged to spend some time in the clinic's chapel. No matter what the patient's religious beliefs may be, the clinic encourages him or her to be at peace spiritually and to make a connection with the Creator.

Hufeland is unique among the German cancer clinics in that it has a Catholic chapel with the Blessed Sacrament reserved in the tabernacle. Patients of all faiths use this chapel to pray and meditate according to their beliefs and practices. Hufeland bought the building from a Catholic organization that stipulated that the Catholic chapel must be maintained and that the head doctor must be a Catholic. Dr. Demuth is Catholic.

Dr. Demuth and his dedicated staff warmly welcome patients of all faiths and cultures from all over the world.

Cost of treatment at the Hufeland Klinik

The Hufeland Klinik's weekly charge of 4,500 Euros includes just about everything:

- Hufeland's medical services
- Chemo or mistletoe if needed
- Room and board for the patient and the patient's companion
- Free shuttle service to and from Frankfurt International Airport

Hufeland recommends a stay of four to six weeks. The cost of four weeks is 17,500 Euros, and the cost of six weeks is 25,500 (slightly less than the 4,500 weekly rate). A follow-up visit is recommended after six months.

Patient feedback about Hufeland

I sent out an e-mail to everyone who bought the first edition of *German Cancer Breakthrough*, requesting feedback – positive or negative – from customers who actually went to one of the clinics I recommended. Six customers gave me feedback about Hufeland. They were all positive.

For example, Kris from Orlando, Florida, wrote, "Wonderful choice for me!" And David from England wrote, "We think the Hufeland clinic is excellent."

Chuck from Arizona sent a dramatic testimonial. He wrote, "I had brain surgery on September 29th for removal of a malignant tumor, which turned out to be glioblastoma multiforme stage 4. I was starting to go downhill and I had trouble forming words, lost my sense of taste, had headaches, couldn't stay awake and my balance was iffy. After the first week at Hufeland my energy came back and all the other symptoms disappeared. I have been home now for two weeks and I am feeling fine. My friends and family say I don't look any different than I ever did and I'm actually back to work."

The kind of brain cancer Chuck had, glioblastoma multiforme, is considered the deadliest, most aggressive form. This cancer would have pulled him under quickly without the German therapies he got at Hufeland.

How to find an open-minded American doctor for follow-up care

If you go to Germany for cancer treatment, it's a good idea to find an open-minded American doctor who can give you follow-up care, such as a monthly infusion of vitamin C by IV for health maintenance. Finding a good doctor in America is especially important for patients who can't afford to make repeat follow-up trips to Germany.

But how do you find such an American doctor who's open to alternatives and who can give you the maintenance treatments to keep cancer from sneaking back?

Probably the easiest way to find a cooperative American physician is to visit the website of the American College for Advancement in Medicine (ACAM): www.acam.org.

From this website you can get a list describing the ACAM doctors in your area by entering your ZIP code.

Hufeland's cancer prevention program

Because it's easier and less expensive to prevent cancer than to cure it, Hufeland now offers a unique five-day cancer prevention package. The program's purpose is not only to prevent cancer but also to boost your health, detox your body, and educate you about a healthy lifestyle.

This program includes a comprehensive review of your medical history, diagnostic procedures such as ultrasound, blood analysis, ECG, a lung function test, tests for three tumor markers, a detox infusion and other health-boosting infusions, five special injections, two ozone treatments, magnetic field therapy, color therapy, reflexology therapy, education about healthy lifestyle choices, and a private consultation with the doctor about test results and potential follow-up treatments.

Here's how the program works. You arrive on a Sunday, and the program begins on Monday. You depart on Friday. At this writing, the price, which includes free pickup from the Frankfurt airport, is 3,900 Euros. This price also includes room and board with the organic Hufeland eating plan for five nights including breakfast, lunch, and dinner. A companion may accompany you in a double room for an extra 75 Euros per night, board and lodging included.

If you're concerned that you might eventually get cancer, you should seriously consider this cancer prevention program.

How to get to the Hufeland Klinik

The nearest major airport is Frankfurt, a two-hour drive from Bad Mergentheim. Hufeland picks up cancer patients for free from this airport.

You may want to rent a car to visit some of the interesting towns in the area, such as Rothenburg, Bayreuth, and Baden-Baden. If you rent a car, it's advisable to stay out of the fast lane, where speed demons sometimes drive well over 100 miles per hour. You'll have no problem driving in the middle lane.

Nearby Rothenburg is the best-preserved medieval walled city in Germany. Its building codes, the strictest in Germany, prevent any modernization. It remains frozen in the 15th century – and it's a magical experience.

Bayreuth, with its annual music festival, is the town made famous by Richard Wagner, the greatest operatic genius of all time. Frau Woeppel told me she has attended a Wagner opera at the Bayreuth festival.

Baden-Baden – the most famous spa town of all – is justly renowned for its historic baths, massages, and saunas. It's about three hours by car from Hufeland.

If you rent a car, be sure to get a navigation system. The car rental agency will show you how to use it, and you can ask the agent to enter the clinic's address into the navigation system. That will make it easy to find the clinic. I bring my own GPS unit to Germany, because I have confidence in it and I'm used to using it.

For extra support Hufeland encourages the patient to bring a spouse or another family member or friend.

After visiting Hufeland, I agree with the patient who said there's something about the "healing energy" in Bad Mergentheim, a charming and historic town.

Contact information:

Hufeland Klinik

Löffelstelzer Straße 1-3 ("ß" is the German symbol for "ss.")
D-97980 Bad Mergentheim, Germany

Website: http://www.hufeland.com (click on the icon of the British flag icon for English)

e-mail: info@hufeland.com

Phone: 011-49-7931-536-0

Fax: 011-49-7931-536-333

Chapter Seven

Dr. Alexander Herzog's Fachklinik in Bad Salzhausen

Just a month before I first toured his clinic in Germany I met Dr. Alexander Herzog at Universal City in Southern California. Dr. Herzog was in Universal City at the invitation of the Cancer Control Society to address its annual convention.

Dr. Herzog's talk was brilliant and articulate. He explained how he applies the most effective alternative and conventional therapies to get the best result for the cancer patient. He highlighted mistletoe therapy and hyperthermia combined with a low dose of chemotherapy. He presented difficult cases of "terminal" cancers that he'd reversed with these therapies, thus proving the therapies' effectiveness.

At the end of his speech, the audience erupted into enthusiastic applause.

Medicine in America would take a giant step forward if every American cancer doctor could hear Dr. Herzog's life-saving, hopeful message. He's a walking encyclopedia of knowledge about the most effective cancer treatments, which have virtually no negative side effects.

On my first visit, I arrived at Dr. Herzog's clinic late in the evening and stayed in one of the rooms there. He was out of town, but I expected to meet with him when he returned the next day.

Dr. Herzog's "Fachklinik" means "Specialty Hospital" in German. The clinic is in a beautiful setting, surrounded by wooded hills, open fields, and meadows. It's a hiker's paradise. The room I stayed in was clean and comfortable. Each patient gets a lot of attention because there are four doctors and 11 nurses. There are 25 beds in the clinic.

Patients come to the Fachklinik from all over the world: Russia, Cameroon, Hungary, Canada, Greece, America, the Middle East, Australia, and elsewhere – from 76 countries so far.

The clinic's chef prepared me an excellent breakfast, which I enjoyed in the cheerful, friendly atmosphere of the cafeteria. Some English-speaking people were seated at the next table. I introduced myself and learned they were part of a family from Canada whose little boy was there for cancer treatment. Without hesitation they gave Dr. Herzog's clinic the thumbs up.

It's worth noting that Dr. Herzog's clinic accepts children; some clinics don't.

At breakfast, I also talked to a man of Dutch ancestry from South Africa who was well pleased with his treatment at the Fachklinik.

Later in the morning I took a stroll in Bad Salzhausen's spa park, just a half-block down the street from the clinic. The park features a functioning antique waterwheel, a band shell with a seating area for outdoor concerts, walking paths, and several springs. I sampled the water from two of the springs.

The water from the Lithiumquelle had a surprisingly strong, heavily mineralized taste that's hard to describe. It wasn't disgusting, just heavy and thick. It's not what you're expecting when you take a sip from a drinking fountain. Dr. Herzog particularly recommends that patients drink the water from this spring because it supports the production of white blood cells.

The water from the Södergrundquelle next to the band shell, on the other hand, had a distinctly salty taste. A plaque next to each fountain lists the specific mineral content.

Because time ran short, I wasn't able to personally visit the actual spa facilities (the pool, etc.) at Bad Salzhausen, even though they are located just a stone's throw from Dr. Herzog's clinic.

By the way, Bad Salzhausen isn't listed on road maps. The name of the city is Nidda, and Bad Salzhausen is simply a spa park near Nidda. There are several other clinics in Bad Salzhausen besides Dr. Herzog's Fachklinik, but Dr. Herzog's is the only cancer clinic.

When Dr. Herzog got back to the clinic, he first had to attend to his patients. I met him after lunch.

Scientific proof is important, says Dr. Herzog

Dr. Herzog personally escorted me through his clinic. He said, "Scientific research is important because you have to prove that what you're doing has a benefit for the patient. If you're not able to prove it, everybody will doubt it."

He meticulously assembled his proof – which consisted of case studies – and presented it to the 23rd annual meeting of the European Society for Hyperthermic Oncology, an organization that focuses on treating cancer through hyperthermia.

The Fachklinik handles the full range of cancers except cases of acute leukemia, which require special treatments. Dr. Herzog can give an appropriate referral to patients with acute leukemia. Dr. Herzog wants the patient to have the *best possible care*, and he'll refer the patient elsewhere if he feels another clinic can do a better job.

As Dr. Herzog said, "Sometimes I tell a prospective patient, 'The best isn't here. Go there.' It's important that doctors cooperate."

Dr. Herzog is a grand master of hyperthermia. He utilizes three kinds of whole-body hyperthermia:

- Moderate hyperthermia, in which the patient's core temperature is raised to 101-103 degrees Fahrenheit for two hours, which simulates a natural fever.
- Systemic hyperthermia, which raises the core temperature to 105 degrees F.
- Extreme hyperthermia, which goes up to 107 degrees F., as Dr. Herzog practices it.

Dr. Herzog is one of the few physicians in the world with the equipment, training, and experience to deploy all three kinds of hyperthermia as appropriate. For many patients, Dr. Herzog uses a low dose of chemotherapy when the patient's body temperature reaches the desired plateau. He says that's when cancer cells are most sensitive to the chemo.

But for some patients, Dr. Herzog uses whole-body hyperthermia without any chemotherapy.

He told us it's not a simple matter to operate the machine. You have to know what you're doing. His experience is vast: over 4,000 treatments of whole-body hyperthermia.

During whole-body hyperthermia, the patient's vital signs are closely monitored. Dr. Herzog says that the patient loses five kilograms of weight through perspiration during hyperthermia. That's 11 pounds! And that's why it's necessary to give the patient five liters of fluid (about 11 pints – a pint weighs a pound) through an IV drip during the hyperthermia. It's essential to keep the patient hydrated because the kidneys must be working (able to flush) for chemo to work.

Harsh side effects? "Absolutely not!"

I asked Dr. Herzog, "Are there any harsh side effects to the hyperthermia or chemotherapy?"

Without hesitation, he replied, "No. Absolutely not." And I wish every American cancer doctor could hear what Dr. Herzog told me next:

"Our principle is that the treatment itself shouldn't harm the patient more than the disease already does. That means if the patient has more problems after the treatment, we're doing something wrong. That's important. We want to have success in terms of killing the cancer cells but we don't want to kill the patient with the treatment. It doesn't make any sense to have 'success' with the treatment that results in a dead patient. Some doctors literally treat patients to death."

It's refreshing to hear such wisdom and common sense.

The machine Dr. Herzog uses for the three different types of whole-body hyperthermia is the very same model used at the university hospitals in Munich and Berlin. It's incredibly sophisticated, with a price tag of about 200,000 Euros.

Dr. Herzog says, "During hyperthermia the patient gets the medication while sleeping. He doesn't feel the treatment or the chemo, which is administered through an IV drip. He sleeps, and by the time he wakes up the treatment is over."

To kill the cancer cells with hyperthermia and low-dose chemo, Dr. Herzog explained, "we have to strengthen the immune system." He accomplishes that through a variety of therapies such as mistletoe, thymus peptides, vitamin C by IV, magnetic-field therapy, ozone therapy, and oxygen therapy.

He also administers fever therapy by injection.

Dr. Herzog demonstrates his magnetic-field therapy machine

When Dr. Herzog showed me his magnetic-field machine, he turned it on and pointed out that you can't *see* that anything is happening. But he placed a couple of small metallic objects in the palm of my hand and told me to put it into the magnetic field. The metallic objects began to shake and vibrate, proving beyond a doubt that his machine produced a strong magnetic energy field.

Dr. Herzog said that magnetic-field therapy increases circulation and supports healing processes of all kinds. He added that studies from the University of Heidelberg prove that fractures and other kinds of injury heal faster with magnetic-field therapy.

Many patients buy their own magnetic-field therapy device and use it in the privacy of their homes to boost the immune system, improve circulation, promote better oxygenation throughout the bodies, and get more pep.

Why Dr. Herzog's clinic is safe from dangerous hospital "bugs"

Dr. Herzog is justifiably proud of his facility. It doesn't have the look or smell of a clinic, and this is important for improving the patient's outlook. Some people actually vomit when they think of going to a hospital, because of bad experiences they've had.

With confidence, Dr. Herzog said he has no hospital "bugs" such as staph and strep – the kind of bugs that spread so easily in conventional hospitals. Dr. Herzog said, "This isn't a problem at the Fachklinik because we have no septic surgical theater." Therefore, without an operating room, there's a minimal risk of bad bugs at the clinic.

And even if someone were to bring a bad bug in from outside, it wouldn't be able to spread. That's because there's no centralized ventilation or ductwork to spread the bugs.

Dr. Herzog's clinic has an impressive program to address the patient's soul, including music therapy and art therapy. As he said, "Patients develop artistic skills here. Many of them have never done anything like that before. They build something, make a sculpture, paint. It helps to avoid stress. It helps to do something *completely different*." One former patient who had never done art before is now selling her own paintings at art exhibitions.

Many patients come to Dr. Herzog's clinic with negative thinking. If another doctor has given a patient a death sentence, Dr. Herzog tells the patient that the doctor isn't God. No doctor can predict how long a patient will live. What encourages such patients is meeting other patients who were given a bad diagnosis but are doing well at the clinic.

Dr. Herzog told me, "Medicine isn't only a science. It's an art. The doctor can give the patient hope; that's half the battle. No doctor should give the patient a bad prognosis.

"Patients in a typical hospital are isolated. It's like being in a prison. They eat in their rooms without socializing with others. That's not the way it is here. Our patients go to the dining room and have meals together. It's a cheerful place. We have organic food, juicing machines, and vegetable and fruit juices. They joke around together. That's important!

"There's no law that patients in a hospital have to eat in their rooms. Hospitals do that probably because that's what they've always done. Our patients can go to the park, walk around, swim at the Therme. They can go sightseeing on the weekend on our bus to Giessen or to Frankfurt for shopping therapy."

The clinic's chapel includes a crucifix, Eastern Orthodox icons, and the Holy Bible. To accommodate Muslim patients, the chapel also includes a Koran and a prayer rug.

In addition to the chapel, the clinic provides patients with a meditation room. Dr. Herzog says the clinic's counselor helps the patient develop strategies against fear and for solving conflicts and stress.

Dr. Herzog's clinic is literally fit for royalty!

Dr. Herzog proudly showed me a picture of Princess Haja of Jordan at the clinic. He said, "She came to support us." Apparently Princess Haja is a fan of the Fachklinik and an admirer of Dr. Herzog.

One of the things patients like about the clinic is the spacious exercise room, which has all kinds of exercise equipment, including a tread mill, weights (dumbbells and barbells), a chin-up bar, an exercise ball, juggling pins, a rebounder, and a punching bag.

This 30-year-old man had given up

I observed one young man in the exercise room doing a vigorous workout. Later I found out that this 30-year-old patient from Oman had come to the clinic short of breath and breathing from an oxygen tank because he had lung cancer from top to bottom. He was desperate, hopeless, and expecting to die soon. When I saw him he had only been at the clinic for about 10 days, but it was obvious that he had his lung power back. What a dramatic recovery! Diagnostics at the University of Giessen revealed that this young man's disease had been misdiagnosed in Oman.

The punching bag can help patients blow off steam, releasing anger and stress. The rebounder is one of those circular mini-trampolines about three feet in diameter. Ten minutes of jumping on the rebounder effectively flushes the body's lymphatic system, a key part of the immune system. When jumping on the rebounder it's not necessary to "get air" by jumping high off the trampoline: gentle jumps in which your feet maintain contact with the mat are enough. Unlike the circulatory system, the lymphatic system lacks a pump to move the lymphatic fluid.

The lymphatic system is normally flushed through exercise, but a good lymphatic massage can also do the job. And that's why patients at the Fachklinik receive lymphatic massage.

The clinic also provides foot reflexology (therapeutic massage of the feet) as well as acupuncture, acupressure, therapeutic baths (hydrotherapy), and homeopathy.

Colonic hydrotherapy is another key therapy. One thing is certain for cancer patients: a gunked-up colon must be thoroughly cleansed to assist the healing process. This normally requires a series of colonic hydrotherapy sessions. One colonic might not be enough.

Health benefits of the local spa

Dr. Herzog pointed out that swimming is available for patients who want to swim: the spa is just a stone's throw away from the clinic. Many patients like to swim, and it's good exercise. But Dr. Herzog says it's far better to *drink* the heavily mineralized waters, because the penetration of minerals through the skin is negligible.

I asked Dr. Herzog about the health benefits of drinking the mineral water. He replied, "It's a question of belief. There are some healing effects, but they've never been studied. People have reported for years that the waters have healing effects."

Dr. Herzog told me about a special place in the spa park, the 100-year-old "inhalatorium," in which mineralized water runs down a wall, creating a kind of humid air that's good for any kind of lung problem. It's a natural method of healing.

For the patient's comfort, relaxation, and pleasure, Dr. Herzog has created two garden patios, one of which has a fish pond. There are so many flowers that two gardeners are necessary to maintain the gardens. One patio is warm in the morning and shaded in the afternoon, and the other is the opposite. So during the warmer months, the patients always have a pleasant place to relax and listen to the birds chirping outside.

Patients who bring their own laptop computer, tablet, or smartphone can access wireless Internet throughout the clinic.

Dr. Herzog's cancer success stories meet the gold standard of proof

When I asked Dr. Herzog to tell me some success stories of patients who'd come to his clinic with "terminal" cancers, without hesitation he reached for his thick scrapbook of success stories. And he pointed out that some of his cases are published in medical journals, which are the gold standard of proof.

As he'd said at the beginning of the interview, "Unless you prove what you're saying, no one will believe you."

57-year-old golfer and marathon runner beats colon and lung cancer

Opening his enormous scrapbook, Dr. Herzog told me about Karl, a 57-year-old pilot, who suffered from colon cancer with metastasis to the lung. He had gone through conventional treatment and was coughing blood – a really bad sign. He'd run marathons and enjoyed golf, but cancer brought his running and golfing to a screeching halt.

Dr. Herzog's treatment included whole-body hyperthermia with a low dose of the 5FU chemotherapy drug. Three months later the metastasis was almost gone, and Karl could run 10 miles per day and play golf. He especially enjoys golfing at his home in Florida.

The British lady who could've suffocated to death

Turning to another page in his scrapbook, Dr. Herzog told me about Andrea, a 44-year-old British lady, who had sarcoma of the right leg with metastasis to the lung. This was a big problem because she could have died from not being able to get enough air. With a tumor in her leg and with her breathing difficulties, she could no longer walk.

Andrea's disease was complicated and required skillful treatment. Dr. Herzog consulted other colleagues, including Professor Thomas

Vogl of the University of Frankfurt, in order to put together the best possible treatment plan for her.

Along with his other therapies, Dr. Herzog used a low dose of chemotherapy, which he fed directly into the tumor through a catheter along with local hyperthermia directly applied to the tumor. To solve the metastasis to the lung, he gave Andrea extreme whole body hyperthermia with low-dose chemo.

This resourceful treatment plan caused the lung metastasis and the tumor to go away. Today Andrea can breathe freely. She's still cancer free.

How 45-year-old Vida beat a big tumor in her lungs

Flipping to another page in his scrapbook, Dr. Herzog told me the story of Vida, a 45-year-old British lady, who came to Dr. Herzog's clinic with a large tumor in her lungs. This form of cancer is particularly dangerous. She underwent Dr. Herzog's treatments, including whole-body hyperthermia. After six weeks the tumor was gone, and she's still free of disease.

Dr. Herzog said, "It's rare for lung cancer to completely heal. I can't promise that to patients, but sometimes it happens."

Woman with facial cancer had drastic surgery, but cancer came back

Turning another page, Dr. Herzog told us about "Mrs. E.," a 41-year-old German woman, with a large tumor in her cheek. She had undergone surgery that removed half of her jaw, followed by good cosmetic reconstructive surgery. But the tumor came back.

In desperation, this lady came to the Fachklinik. Her treatment plan included local hyperthermia with a low dose of 5FU chemo. Dr. Herzog split the hyperthermia in a way he calls "chronomodulated treatment overnight." That means he gave the treatment between 2:00 a.m. and 6:00 a.m. Dr. Herzog told me, "Between 2:00 a.m. and 6:00 a.m. you have less side effects. During the night, the normal cells would rather sleep but the tumor cells are active."

The treatment was effective, and today "Mrs. E." is still in remission.

In 2007 another lady was diagnosed with breast cancer. She had a lump on the left side, which she treated with homeopathy and the "black salve." The treatments didn't work. In December of 2008 she came to Dr. Herzog in desperation. The tumor smelled, and it looked horrible. Dr. Herzog gave her low-dose chemo with hyperthermia and other treatments. Within three months, the tumor was gone. She never had surgery at all.

A Canadian lady came to Dr. Herzog with a lump in her right breast. The tumor was large. Her favorite hobby was dancing, but osteoarthritis had destroyed her hips. In addition to Dr. Herzog's anti-cancer therapies, his cooperating surgeon gave her some surgery, and she got hip replacements. She went back on the dance floor at the age of 76.

A Canadian stewardess came to Dr. Herzog with a lump in her left breast. She shunned conventional therapy and tried some alternative treatments in Canada. But the tumor got worse. It turned into a disaster. Dr. Herzog helped her get rid of the cancer with hyperthermia and low-dose chemo. She suffered no hair loss or other side effects.

65-year-old man beats lymphoma with *no* chemo

My time with Dr. Herzog was up, but he told me one more story. A 65-year-old German, "Mr. L.," came to the clinic with lymphoma. Because the lymphoma was pressing on his bladder, he had to urinate frequently. Dr. Herzog tried to persuade him to use some low-dose chemo, but he refused. He didn't want *any* chemo.

And so Dr. Herzog built a treatment plan with *no* chemo. The treatments, which included homeopathy and local hyperthermia, solved the problem. The lymphoma completely went away, and today Mr. L. is fine.

Certainly Dr. Herzog was born to be a physician. He told me that when he was 12 years old he knew he wanted to be a doctor.

When Dr. Herzog first started out, every cancer patient got pretty much the same treatment. Not any more. He told me that new drugs are now available – targeted drugs – that can benefit some patients. Patients who have lung cancer or melanoma, for example, can benefit from specific treatments.

Dr. Herzog told me that there has been a change in attitude at university hospitals and in the big medical journals: complementary therapy is now "in." They are now open to mistletoe therapy and other complementary and natural therapies, and many are eager to learn about complementary medicine. In fact, Dr. Herzog is also a professor at the University of Giessen, where he teaches complementary therapies in oncology. His students are eager to learn because they want to be able to give answers to their patients in the future.

Dr. Herzog well recognizes that chemo often has more disadvantages than advantages. That's why he only uses it when necessary, and he uses holistic treatments to lessen the side effects, and he also gives the patient detox and immune-boosting therapies after chemo. He said, "Hodgkins and testicular cancer can be cured with chemo: it would be really stupid not to use it in those cases. But in the case of advanced pancreatic or lung cancer, chemo doesn't make sense."

When chemo is warranted, he gives 60 to 70 percent of the standard dose of chemo because he considers the full dose too toxic and unnecessary. His patients have negligible side effects. Some of his Australian patients have continued receiving the same amount of chemo when they returned to Australia and are surprised to experience bad side effects. They ask Dr. Herzog, "Where you really giving me chemo in Germany?" Yes, he was. The Australian doctors who gave the same amount of chemo didn't give the holistic therapies that practically make side effects disappear.

Here are some facts that might interest you:

- Dr. Herzog is a scholar of languages. One day he had patients from England, Spain, France, Germany, and Greece. As he made his rounds visiting each patient, he spoke English, Spanish, French, German, and Greek!

- The spa park across the street has *seven* springs. Each spring originates from a different level under the ground, and each one has a different taste and mineral content. Dr. Herzog said, "Some of them taste bad. The sulphur one smells. But they're all beneficial to drink."

- For the comfort and convenience of the patient, Dr. Herzog can install a port system for access to the bloodstream. That way, it's not necessary to poke around to find a vein.

- In ozone therapy, Dr. Herzog takes out 200 milliliters of blood, mixes the blood with ozone gas (a form of oxygen), shakes the blood, and returns it to the body.

- To meet the spiritual needs of the patients, a Catholic priest and a Protestant minister visit the clinic once a week.

- Dr. Herzog's whole-body hyperthermia machine requires an astounding 3,000 gallons of water for one treatment. (Fortunately, water is plentiful in Germany.) The water filters the irradiation to create a *mild* heat, which doesn't seem hot at all, just warm. But this warmth penetrates *deeply*. The heat goes through the skin and heats up the blood until the patient's body core reaches the desired temperature – even as high as 107 degrees Fahrenheit in extreme hyperthermia.

- He uses a lab in Heidelberg for chemo sensitivity testing to find out which treatments may work and which ones definitely won't work. The tests help him match the patient's cancer cells to the chemotherapeutic drug most likely to be effective against that type of cancer.

- Dr. Herzog gives a lung function test to measure lung capacity. He encourages those patients who are able to give their lungs a workout in the exercise room or outside in the fresh air.

- The Fachklinik sponsors a local cycling team. Dr. Herzog proudly told me that his team is winning championships.

What patients say about Dr. Herzog's Fachklinik

I sent out an e-mail to everyone who bought the first edition of *German Cancer Breakthrough*, requesting feedback – positive or negative – from readers who actually went to one of the clinics I recommended. Ten customers gave me feedback about Dr. Herzog – all of them positive.

For example, Dr. Arnoldo Velloso da Costa has a nutritional practice in Brazil. After reading *German Cancer Breakthrough*, he started referring his cancer patients to Germany. Dr. da Costa wrote, "I found a very good assistance at the Fachklinik directed by Dr Alexander Herzog. I had five successful cases treated there."

Louise from Canada wrote, "The staff, Dr. Herzog and his doctors, nurses etc. were all wonderful and couldn't do enough for you. It was as enjoyable an experience as one could have, given the circumstances."

Peter from Australia: "Your book has saved the life of one of my close friends. She had renal cancer with metastasis everywhere and was given only three months to live."

Neil, an American with homes in New Hampshire and Florida, wrote: "I narrowed my search down to three clinics but ended up choosing the Herzog clinic because of the direct communication I had with Dr. Herzog himself and the very practical treatment protocol he had designed for my particular situation. I couldn't be happier with the choice.

"The staff is highly professional with a personal touch. Dr. Herzog makes a point of visiting personally on a daily basis. This is one of the advantages of being in a small clinic.

"One of the surprises is that I have had to go back for follow-up treatment so many times. I have since found this is typical of most patients. Anyone going to the German clinics has to be prepared for the cost of so many visits and the hassle of airline travel. In my opinion it is worth the effort. We have been surprised to find that Blue Cross/Blue Shield has reimbursed us for about 50% of the cost of the hospital treatments."

This last statement is worth noting. If you have health insurance, you should definitely try to get as much reimbursement as you can. See chapter sixteen of this book: "How to raise funds or get insurance reimbursement for your cancer treatment in Germany."

What if you can't afford multiple trips for follow-up care?

Neil's comment about repeat trips concerns me because many people can't afford to make multiple trips to Germany. Those who can only afford to make one or two trips can do a couple of things to keep their cancer from sneaking back: (1) Read, re-read, and apply the ideas in the chapter "Cancer dilemma: Do you swat mosquitoes or drain the swamp?" Making the necessary lifestyle changes can keep the odds tipped in your favor. (2) One long-term brain cancer survivor who got rid of his cancer in Germany was able to obtain a vitamin C IV treatment every month in America. Nothing succeeds like success, and this is an affordable maintenance therapy that's worth considering.

To get maintenance therapies like vitamin C by IV in America, you'll need an open-minded physician. You can find one near you through the American College for Advancement in Medicine (ACAM). Simply log onto ACAM's website and enter your ZIP code. The website is www.acam. org.

American patient questions a German tradition

After ordering *German Cancer Breakthrough,* Tom from Tennessee went to Dr. Herzog's clinic for treatment. Here's what Tom wrote to me about his experience: "Dr. Herzog is a wonderful person, caring and compassionate, and he appears very knowledgeable about oncology and hyperthermia. His treatment worked."

But Tom questioned some of the food choices available in the dining room. He said, "It's odd that they have cake and coffee every afternoon at a cancer clinic, but it's a German tradition. The food is good but not what you'd expect from an 'alternative' doctor – pork, beef, cheese, sweets, etc. They did have a juicer that all of us used every day."

Tom is right in saying that cake and coffee in the afternoon is a German tradition – much like 4:00 tea in England. And Dr. Herzog's clinic isn't the only alternative cancer clinic that observes this tradition.

Here's what Dr. Herzog told me about diet, "We offer food adapted to the needs of cancer patients. Fresh, organic produce. Fruits and vegetables. We have a juicing machine, and patients press their own fresh juice. It's important to get fruits and vegetables. With pancreatic cancer, the patient can't digest the ideal anti-cancer diet because the stomach and bowels don't work right. They need special foods adapted to their limitations.

"We discuss anti-cancer diets: macrobiotic, Gerson, and so on. Not one diet has shown that it really works. Patients who don't eat anything are miserable! Some diets don't allow any coffee, wine, bread, cheese, nothing. We're a bit more open. If someone eats an ice cream or a piece of cake, cancer won't immediately grow because they ate it. It's not that serious if you have an ice cream or a piece of cake. A strict diet isn't necessary. The Mediterranean diet is the best one. In Italy and southern France they eat pasta, small portions of meat, freshly prepared vegetables, olive oil, wine, tiramisu, baguettes, and apple cake. And they have 30 percent less cancer. It's not really a 'diet' because you can eat good things.

"Some grains can't be digested by patients with pancreatic cancer. The diet should be sensible so the patient knows what's important. Patients shouldn't eat too much and should lose weight if they're overweight."

As for exercise, Dr. Herzog says running a marathon is too extreme. He advises this instead: "If you have a daily activity program for 30 minutes – a brisk walk, garden work, yoga, or dancing – do that regularly, and you'll have a better prognosis. Exercise can be as good as medicine but much cheaper."

Because of Dr. Herzog's credentials, experience, track record, and positive feedback from his patients, I continue to recommend his clinic.

Cost of treatment at Dr. Herzog's Fachklinik

Treatment at the Fachklinik costs about 6,000 Euros per week, including hyperthermia, and the average stay is two to three weeks. Dr. Herzog emphasizes that cancer is a chronic disease that requires permanent lifestyle changes as well as long-term care and follow up.

Patients normally come with a friend or relative, and the clinic charges a modest fee of 46 Euros a day for room and board for the relative.

How to get to the Fachklinik

Getting to the Fachklinik is easy. You just fly into Frankfurt, and the clinic will send someone to pick you up free of charge. It's that simple!

But if you want to explore the surrounding area, you may choose to rent a car. You'll easily be able to make day trips to such exciting and enjoyable places as Rothenburg (Germany's best-preserved walled city) and Bayreuth (famous for its Wagner music festival).

Contact information:

Fachklinik Dr. Herzog (Specialty Hospital Dr. Herzog)

Kurstraße 16-18
D-63667 Nidda, Germany

Contact: Dr. A. Herzog

Website: www.fachklinikdrherzog.de

e-mail: info@hospitaldrherzog.de

Phone: 011-49-6043-983-0

Fax: 011-49-6043-983-194

Chapter Eight

Dr. Friedrich Migeod's BioMed Klinik in Bad Bergzabern

The BioMed Klinik is located amidst vineyards in Germany's charming and picturesque wine region. It's about five miles from the French border and not far from Strasbourg, one of the most romantic cities in Europe.

You'll find the BioMed Klinik in the small town of Bad Bergzabern, famed for its historic cityscape. Bad Bergzabern also has a spa with naturally mineralized waters. Nearby is the ultimate spa town, Baden-Baden. Bad Bergzabern also has a local winery that produces excellent wines, both white and red, for local consumption only.

Patients come to BioMed from countries all over the world, including America, Canada, Australia, Indonesia, and Brazil. Most of the foreign cancer patients have been told their cancer was "hopeless" and "terminal." Doctors back home have told them, "Nothing more can be done." But BioMed doctors tell them, "We'll try." And BioMed's impressive results prove that those conventional doctors are often wrong.

BioMed is a large in-patient clinic. Its two buildings hold an impressive 135 beds. It has an impeccable reputation for professionalism and an impressive record of success. For example, the American whistle-blower and health advocate Dr. Ralph Moss highly recommends this clinic.

Five-year-old boy with brain cancer *enjoys* his treatments!

During one of my visits to BioMed I interviewed Michala from Greece. She was glad to let me interview her.

Michala wasn't at the clinic for herself. Rather, she was there for a follow-up visit with her 5-year-old son, Socrates. Her cheerful little boy had been diagnosed a year-and-a-half earlier with perhaps the deadliest form of brain cancer, glioblastoma multiforme.

Conventional doctors consider this kind of brain cancer a death sentence, and the conventional treatments for children are harsh. The cancer (or the conventional treatment) usually kills children within a year.

Because Socrates was doing well a year and a half after his diagnosis, he had already enjoyed a six-month bonus. And best of all, says his mother, he enjoys an outstanding quality of life because there are no side effects to BioMed's treatments.

Visualize how a child with brain cancer would react when his parents bring him back to a conventional hospital for another round of conventional treatment. Recalling the misery caused by the previous round, the child would be kicking and screaming in terror.

But it's nothing like that at BioMed!

Little Socrates wasn't one bit afraid to re-enter BioMed for the follow-up visit. Michala said that he thinks it's sort of like they're staying in a hotel on vacation. And in between the treatments Michala takes Socrates out for fun side-trips, just as if they were on vacation.

Michala knows from personal experience what children with brain cancer suffer in hospital cancer wards in Athens. The high toxicity of the treatments makes them lose their hair and their color. It's heartbreaking that conventional doctors subject so many children to this kind of misery.

In Greece, when Socrates first came down with brain cancer, his parents followed the doctors' advice and plugged him into conventional treatment. And so he underwent surgery, radiation, and chemo for three months.

When the tumor came back, a doctor advised them: "Go home. Don't take any therapy." The doctor just gave up and recommended that the parents do the same. But they didn't take that death sentence as the last word.

Instead, they looked for an alternative. Other doctors said, "There's nothing we can do." His parents kept looking.

Some people in Greece recommended BioMed because of its impressive track record of treating tough and stubborn brain cancers.

When Michala contacted BioMed, they didn't say no, though they normally don't accept children. They said, "We'll try." Michala told me, "BioMed is a very good choice."

Though Michala said it's not easy to deal with the stress of having a child with brain cancer, she added, "When we're here we go to the Schwarzwald (the Black Forest). We go to the lake. We meet other people. Staying at the typical cancer hospital is like staying in a prison. That's not the way it is here. This is a good way of life. This is a good benefit."

Effective cancer treatments don't have to be pure hell

Indeed, BioMed, like all the other clinics I visited, doesn't look or smell at all like a hospital. And the cancer treatments are mild, not harsh.

I watched little Socrates playing happily on the floor with his toys. He was as cheerful as any other boy his age. It's *disgraceful* that so many hospitals in the USA needlessly put children with cancer through *hell*. When will this cruel medical insanity in America end?

At first, BioMed's Medical Director told Michala that he didn't want to give Socrates any chemotherapy. Later he recommended *some*

chemo, but only a low dose. It hasn't caused the boy any problems.

Michala said they were in BioMed when her son's fifth birthday rolled around. The secretaries, nurses, and other staff members gave him presents. They held a big party with a lot of balloons and a big cake. He had a wonderful birthday.

As Michala explained, "Here at BioMed it's as if everyone has given us a big hug. Everybody treats Socrates with love. Greek people are loud, and Germans are quiet. But nobody complains about us. The staff is always helpful. Socrates is a good friend of the ladies who clean the room. Every morning they bring him a toy and play games with him."

BioMed's head psychologist Erika told me, "Socrates is at the point where psychotherapy can really make the difference between life and death. Socrates enjoys living. For a cancer patient, that's important. If life isn't fun, some cancer patients just give up." Psychology is an integral part of BioMed's treatment plan.

Three years later I heard that Socrates was still doing fine.

Mild treatments – no harsh side effects

BioMed is the largest hyperthermia center in Europe. Like the other German cancer clinics I visited, BioMed often uses hyperthermia in conjunction with low-dose chemo. Patients suffer no harsh side effects from this mild form of treatment. It's even mild enough for a child – as in the case of Socrates.

Two staff members, receptionist Marit Ehnert and head psychologist Erika Haese, gave me a tour. These two lovely ladies, both of whom speak fluent English, were happy to sit down for an interview.

We asked Marit and Erika to tell me about some patients who'd gotten rid of "terminal" cancer. They obliged.

Former bone cancer patient zips around Europe on a motorcycle

In 1995, a 55-year-old German named Georg (pronounced "Gayorg") came to BioMed as a last resort for his metastasized bone cancer. He had cancer from head to toe. He could barely walk. He went through BioMed's treatment plan, which includes hyperthermia, detoxification, and mistletoe.

Now – twelve years later – he's going on a motorbike tour throughout Europe. He keeps in touch with the staff at BioMed, who saved his life.

Stomach cancer patient gives up on chemo

Dieter, a 42-year-old man from the Frankfurt area, came to BioMed suffering from stomach cancer that had spread to his liver, spleen, and entire abdomen. In Heidelberg he had received chemotherapy, but the chemo had no effect whatsoever on the cancer. His doctors didn't expect him to live.

At BioMed Dieter received a special kind of chemo in low doses along with whole-body hyperthermia. Fourteen years later, he's still doing fine.

Patient from Spain gets rid of metastasized prostate cancer

Conventional doctors could do nothing for Friedrich, a 60-year-old prostate cancer patient living in Spain. His cancer had metastasized and was running amok throughout his body. He came to BioMed and underwent two cycles of hyperthermia with low-dose chemo. Today he remains cancer-free.

The treatment plan at BioMed includes these therapies:

- A healthful low-meat diet emphasizing fruits and vegetables and discouraging sugar
- Detoxification, including colonic hydrotherapy
- Magnetic-field therapy
- Oxygen therapy
- Ozone therapy
- Hyperthermia (sometimes called "fever therapy")
- Dendritic cells
- Psychological counseling and relaxation exercises
- Therapeutic massage
- Qigong exercises that relieve pain
- Mistletoe therapy
- Insulin potentiation therapy (IPT)
- Infrared therapy for skin metastasis
- Light therapy
- Art therapy
- Music therapy

After touring BioMed, Marit suggested I visit the local winery, which I did. I chatted with Stefan Hitziger, the young man who owns the winery. He proudly offered me samples of his wines – both red and white. He doesn't produce enough wine to sell it outside his local market. I bought a bottle of his Gewürztraminer, a delightful white wine – a bargain at five Euros.

Marit also recommended that I try a dish called "saumagen" at a local restaurant. This regional specialty is a favorite of the German statesman Helmut Kohl. Again, I followed her advice to the letter when I went to one of the local restaurants in the historic district. The tasty vegetable and pork dish included a generous mound of sauerkraut.

Dr. Hager published his proof in scientific journals

If you're interested in investigating scientific proof of the effectiveness of BioMed's therapies, you can read the late Dr. Dieter Hager's article "Deep Hyperthermia with Radiofrequencies in Liver Metastases," which was published in the scholarly journal *Anticancer Research* 19: 3403-3408 (1999). Dr. Hager founded BioMed.

In his study, 80 patients were treated for colorectal cancer with liver metastases. They were given hyperthermia and low-dose chemo. The study found that the average survival time was "twice as high as expected" – compared to patients treated with chemotherapy alone.

Dr. Hager also published an article titled "Intraperitoneal hyperthermic perfusion chemotherapy (IPHC) for patients with chemotherapy-resistant peritoneal disseminated ovarian cancer." This study, which involved 36 patients, found that IPHC is associated with a marked prolongation of survival and improvement in quality of life. The reference can be found in the *International Journal of Gynecologic Cancer* 2001;11 (Suppl. 1): 57-63.

In addition, Dr. Hager published scholarly articles about such things as hyperthermia and glioblastoma brain cancer in the German scholarly journal *Deutsche Zeitschrift für Onkologie*, but I'm not aware that they have been translated into English.

How to get to the BioMed Klinik

Americans who want to go to BioMed for treatment first need to send the facts about their case to the clinic. This information is usually sent over the Internet. One of the English-speaking doctors then looks over the records and makes a recommendation.

The patient then makes the flight arrangements. Patients can fly into Frankfurt or Stuttgart.

Patients and their companions usually rent a car and drive to the clinic. That's because most patients like to explore the surrounding area. France is just five miles away, and the historic French city of Strasbourg with its charming blend of French and German culture is a short drive away.

Marit told me that in Strasbourg you can buy a card for 6 Euros that gives you admission to all of Strasbourg's 14 museums. And she said Strasbourg at Christmastime is simply a must – a dazzling fairyland for people of all ages.

If the patient can't rent a car or prefers not to, other ways to get to the clinic are available. The clinic can provide details.

One advantage of staying at BioMed is its proximity to France. If you love France, look no further! BioMed is also near the famous Schwarzwald (Black Forest).

Though I didn't have time to visit the local Therme (the pool and sauna complex), I heard good things about it. It's definitely an advantage to have such a facility close to the clinic. Bad Bergzabern is beautiful and captivating.

Some patients prefer a small, intimate clinic; others prefer a larger clinic. BioMed is quite large (135 beds).

BioMed's medical director, Friedrich Migeod, M.D., used to be on the staff of the Pro Life Klinik in Igls/Innsbruck, Austria, where I first met him. Before that, he was at St. Georg in Bad Aibling working under Friedrich Douwes, M.D. Dr. Migeod certainly has a lot of experience.

He's perhaps the only doctor in the world who's curing liver cancer with a simple, quick, effective procedure called the "hot needle."

Liver cancer patients need the "hot needle"

Dr. Migeod believes that in many cases liver cancer doesn't need surgery. Instead, it needs the "hot needle." He started using the "hot needle" 16 years ago at St. Georg. He was the only one who could do it, and he cured over 300 liver cancer patients at that clinic, including patients who had metastasis to the liver. He has done over 100 "hot needle" cures at BioMed.

To perform the "hot needle" treatment, Dr. Migeod gives the patient a local anesthetic in the liver area. The patient lies on the left side, so no bleeding can occur. While monitoring by way of ultrasound, the doctor puts a special needle right into the middle of the metastatic tumor. Then he heats up the tip of the needle about as much as a lamp, using a mild electric current. The tip of the needle gets hot – 70 degrees, 80 degrees, 90 degrees Celsius – and hot water comes out of the tip of the needle. The cancer cells simply can't take the heat, and die by the millions.

Dr. Migeod told me, "On the ultrasound screen during this procedure, you see a cloud around the area of the needle. When the cloud reaches the boundary of the metastasis, then you know the heat has reached the outer boundary, so you heat up just a little more to be sure you have everything." The procedure lasts about an hour or less, and the patient normally has no pain because the liver has no nerves. Then the doctor removes the needle, and the patient lies on his left side for three or four hours.

The results of this simple, minor procedure are the equivalent of major liver surgery! Dr. Migeod told me, "It works if the metastases aren't too large or too many." If he's still the only doctor in the world who's using the "hot needle," he needs to teach some other doctors how to do it!

Believe it or not, over 100 years ago the *New York Times* featured an article with this headline: "Hot Needle for Cancer" (September 25, 1915). Why is this amazing treatment, which has been around for a century, so little known and so little used?

If a liver cancer patient isn't a candidate for the "hot needle" treatment, Dr. Migeod sends the patient to the University of Frankfurt for a specialized treatment, CT scan with laser, which is highly effective in complicated cases where the metastasis is large. The University of Frankfurt hospital also gives the patient chemo by perfusion directly to the liver. Then the patient returns to BioMed for hyperthermia, which enhances the chemo that's still in the liver from the perfusion therapy.

Another thing I learned from Dr. Migeod is that BioMed is one of the clinics that uses hyperthermic perfusion therapy for peritoneal cancer and also for bladder cancer.

Here's how that therapy works: The peritoneum is the membrane that forms the lining of the abdominal cavity. In hyperthermic perfusion therapy, the doctor uses a dialysis machine to infuse a liquid that's heated to 48 degrees Celsius (118 degrees Fahrenheit) into the peritoneal cavity. One hundred to 200 milliliters of this heated liquid, which can contain a chemo drug, is pumped in and out of the cavity for an hour or two with a local anesthetic. During the procedure the patient relaxes on a bed with a doctor and nurse nearby. The patient feels no burning or discomfort. It's an easy treatment because the chemo is confined to the abdominal area and doesn't circulate throughout the patient's body.

Bladder cancer patients can also benefit from hyperthermic perfusion therapy, in which the heated liquid is pumped in and out of the bladder.

Natural "chemo" for brain cancer

BioMed has developed a combination therapy for brain cancer that Dr. Migeod explained at a medical conference in America in 2009. He presented statistical proof that you can improve the survival of brain cancer patients by adding local hyperthermia and frankincense.

Frankincense has a good effect on brain tumors because it blocks cells that want to duplicate. Dr. Migeod told me, "This has been investigated and verified scientifically. It's like a natural chemo with no side effects." BioMed prefers African frankincense. Brain cancer patients swallow 10 to 15 frankincense capsules a day (four to five grams). Frankincense reduces the water around the tumor. Many of the symptoms are the result of the water around the tumor.

BioMed also uses vitamins D and A for brain cancers. Socrates, the little Greek boy, used these therapies to beat his glioblastoma multiforme.

For adult brain cancer patients, BioMed also prescribes thalidomide. It's non-toxic, and the only side effect is that it makes the patient sleepy, so it should only be taken in the evening. Thalidomide is one of the three methods BioMed uses to shut down the blood vessels that feed the tumor. (The other two methods are hyperthermia and quercetin, a plant-extract supplement.) Thalidomide can help beat the toughest brain cancers, but it must never be taken by pregnant women or women who may become pregnant.

Patients avail themselves of the healing waters of Bad Bergzabern

Bad Bergzabern is a spa town that's famous for mineralized waters that are said to have medicinal value. Patients may, if they like, take advantage of the local "Therme," the complex of therapeutic baths that includes hot pools, cold pools, saunas, and therapeutic massage.

Dr. Migeod said that the patients definitely enjoy and benefit from the local spa park. There's a Kneipp wading pool course in the park. This consists of a row of five or six shallow pools. The Kneipp water therapy helps train the blood vessels, which improves circulation. Some patients make a tour of the pools in the morning. The spa park is only about 300 yards from the clinic. It's a large park — about a mile long. If a patient doesn't feel like walking back up to the clinic from the park, a driver can pick the patient up.

Dr. Migeod said it's possible to do a Kneipp water therapy at home in the shower — alternating between hot and cold water. Another way is to use two buckets of water — one hot and the other cold — and take a foot bath, alternating between the two buckets. If you end the therapy with cold water, it can make you naturally sleepy and improve your sleep.

BioMed's dietary recommendations

BioMed considers nutrition crucial for cancer patients. A well trained chef on the staff prepares all the meals. There's no catering. All the food is fresh and low in carbs.

Patients often ask, "What should I eat? Which supplements should I take?" While one size doesn't fit all, BioMed educates patients about nutrition and cooking. Cancer patients generally need vitamin D supplementation, but the clinic checks the patient's vitamin D level before recommending a supplemental amount. Tomato juice combined with black pepper and curcumin is an excellent antioxidant drink, which BioMed offers its patients. Green tea is also recommended.

Cost of treatment at BioMed

The cost of treatment varies, depending on how long you stay and what kind of treatments you get. Normally, patients spend two weeks at the clinic. Sometimes one week is enough if the case isn't complicated. A stay of 10 to 14 days would cost in the range of 8,000 to 12,000 Euros, depending on the treatments and medication. At the end of your stay a detailed invoice is issued.

There's a nominal charge for companions who want to stay at the clinic. Or they can stay at a local Bed & Breakfast.

Treatment starts on the first day, and treatments take place every day except Sunday. The treatment schedule is intensive. Each patient gets an e-mail describing the treatment plan.

The clinic provides wireless Internet.

Patient feedback about BioMed

During my most recent tour of BioMed, I met a man from Waukegan, Illinois, while he was receiving local hyperthermia for his cancer. Obviously happy with his treatment, he told me he had read *German Cancer Breakthrough*. He said, "You're the reason I'm here!"

I met another patient – Ken, a businessman from Loveland, Colorado – who was also at BioMed as a result of reading *German Cancer Breakthrough*. Ken told me he'd battled difficult health problems for years, including ulcerative colitis and rheumatoid arthritis. Prescription drugs didn't work but compromised his immune system. When his doctor suspected that he also had prostate cancer he wanted to do a biopsy. Ken said no. He came to BioMed not only for prostate treatment but also to get some real help for his autoimmune disease.

Ken told me, "I feel like I'm coming away from here knowing what I'm dealing with and having made some really good progress. With proper monitoring and a good protocol, I'll be all right. These folks here have spent more time with me in two weeks than conventional doctors in America have in years. Everybody has been wonderful. Everybody: the maintenance people, the kitchen people, the nurses. I was taken aback a little bit by just how genuinely interested and nice everybody is. It's hard to find this kind of medical care in America."

I sent out an e-mail to everyone who bought the first edition of *German Cancer Breakthrough*, requesting feedback – positive or negative – from customers who actually went to one of the clinics I recommended. I got feedback about BioMed from a man named Bryce from Canada. Bryce and his father personally toured four of the clinics featured in my book before selecting BioMed. Bryce wrote, "We were very impressed with BioMed and felt that the staff and standard of treatment were of very high calibre. We chose this clinic for my Mom."

Bryce's father, Allan, wrote, "I consider BioMed a quality medical facility with great integrity." I agree with that assessment.

Contact information:

BioMed Klinik

Tischbergerstraße 5 + 8
D-76887 Bad Bergzabern, (

Contact: Mrs. Lehmann

Website: www.biomed-klinik.de

e-mail: info@biomed-klinik.de

Phone: 011-49-6343-705-0

Fax: 011-49-6343-705-928

Chapter Nine

Dr. Thomas Rau's Paracelsus Klinik in Lustmühle, Switzerland

The doctor on the German side of the lake was furious at the cancer doctors on the Swiss side. Unlike the other German doctors I interviewed, this German doctor was like most American cancer doctors. He believed in only three ways to treat cancer: surgery, radiation, and chemo. He was miffed when one of his patients, 62-year-old Barbara from Germany, refused his recommendation of chemotherapy for her breast cancer.

She just said "no" to chemo. She wanted to avoid the misery and side effects. But her doctor couldn't handle the rejection. He wasn't used to patients taking their health into their own hands.

When the doctor found out that Barbara was getting alternative treatments at the Paracelsus cancer clinic across the lake in Switzerland, he hit the ceiling. He fired off a letter to the Paracelsus doctors, threatening to sue them for "irresponsible" treatment. That was in 2004.

Despite the threat of legal action for "irresponsible" treatment, the Paracelsus doctors knew they were on the right track. They were confident they could help Barbara get rid of her cancer without harsh conventional treatments.

Barbara went through the three-week treatment program at Paracelsus, an outpatient clinic that's famous for curing cancer with state-of-the-art natural treatments.

Barbara went back to Germany with a solid plan to keep her cancer from returning. She has been cancer free ever since then. She's happy to return to the Swiss clinic for follow-up visits, and she still gets vitamin C treatments by IV for preventive purposes and to strengthen her health.

Following her astonishing recovery, Barbara had a colonoscopy at a clinic on the German side of the lake. A polyp was removed, but the doctor didn't clamp it right and there was some bleeding. Barbara's surgeon was astounded that she recovered from this slight complication within just one day. Her healing process was almost immediate.

The surgeon was also amazed that she wasn't taking any prescription drugs. Barbara told the surgeon that she was only taking the nutritional supplements that the Paracelsus doctors recommend — no drugs.

Hostile doctor changes his mind about Paracelsus

Even the doctor on the German side of the lake who had earlier threatened Paracelsus with legal action for "irresponsible" treatment has had a change of heart. Every time he sees Barbara, he marvels at how healthy she is. He's now asking Barbara about the natural treatments she got at Paracelsus: "What are they DOING up there?"

"Up there" is literally up there! Paracelsus Klinik is perched above the historic Swiss town of St. Gallen in the Swiss Alps on the southern side of a gigantic alpine lake.

To prepare for my first visit to Paracelsus, which is named after a great Swiss physician of the Renaissance period, I asked the clinic for advice on where to stay. The clinic's patient coordinator Barbara Bischofberger e-mailed me three recommendations. I decided to stay the least-expensive of the three, the Pension Alpenheim Bed and Breakfast in Teufen. It was an excellent value.

My clinic tour guide was the charming young lady I had been in touch with by e-mail, Barbara Bischofberger. As Barbara walked me through the clinic, she told me about the eating plan for cancer patients that the clinic's director Dr. Thomas Rau, M.D., recommends. It's a largely vegetarian eating plan that's low in carbs. This is the same eating plan that's offered to patients who stay at the nearby hotel. I discovered how delicious this food is when I had lunch later that day with Dr. Rau and some of his associates.

Each cancer patient meets with the clinic's nutritionist, Sonja, because the physicians at Paracelsus believe eating the right foods is crucial to cancer recovery.

Monday through Friday the cancer patients are kept busy with eight or nine different treatments each day. The scheduling is well organized. Therapies start at 7:30 a.m. and go until about 5:00 p.m. The clinic is closed on Saturday and Sunday.

Paracelsus offers an impressive array of treatments including:

- Whole body hyperthermia up to 40 degrees Celsius (104 degrees Fahrenheit)
- Local hyperthermia
- Insulin potentiation therapy with low-dose chemo
- Live-cell therapy
- Sanum and Isopathic treatment to change the milieu and remove harmful bacteria and parasites
- Mistletoe therapy
- Lactic acid therapy
- Vitamin C infusions
- Infusions to alkalize the body
- Homeopathic infusions
- EDTA infusions (chelation) to detoxify the body
- Liver detoxification

- Colonic hydrotherapy
- Oxygen therapy
- Ozone therapy
- Pulsed magnetic field therapy to boost the immune system and accelerate healing
- Lymphatic massage for detoxification
- Infrared sauna to detoxify the body through the skin
- Thermography, which measures the body's temperature in various spots. Abnormal heat patterns can identify weaknesses in various organs.
- Darkfield microscopy, a diagnostic tool that allows patients to see their own living blood under high magnification. Patients can actually see their blood becoming healthier during their course of treatment, and that encourages them and promotes healing.
- Cardio-sonic treatments to reactivate the parasympathetic nervous system; through this treatment the patient learns how to regulate the heartbeat, relax, and manage stress.
- Acupuncture
- Cupping — a procedure that uses suction to induce microcirculation. Suction cups are placed along the appropriate meridian, along the back usually. This procedure helps detoxification through the skin by increasing blood flow rate within the minor capillaries of the skin.
- Foot reflexology

Some therapies, such as colonic hydrotherapy and cupping, are given twice a week. Other therapies, especially IV infusions, are given every day, Monday through Friday. Patients take their infusions in one of the infusion rooms such as the Chalet Room or the Quiet Room.

The Quiet Room at Paracelsus is incredible. It's breathtaking. Through huge picture windows I saw cows and sheep grazing in the alpine meadows. I saw flowers everywhere. Though it's called the Quiet Room, it's not completely quiet, because I heard the sound of cowbells from the meadows — a pleasing sound indeed.

To say that Paracelsus is located in a charming part of Switzerland would be an understatement! Another room that particularly impressed me was the Chalet Room with its knotty pine paneling. Patients find the Chalet Room a wonderful place to relax while they're getting their IV infusion therapy.

You can hear the soothing sound of running water from the fountain on the ground floor of Paracelsus because of the building's open architecture. A spiral staircase leads to the upper floors.

What's extraordinary about Paracelsus is that it has just about everything you need to cure cancer — even a biological dentistry department — under one roof ! Well, two roofs, actually. There are two adjacent buildings: the dental building and the main building. During the tour I was amazed at the vast array of cancer treatments offered. Indeed, Dr. Rau later told me that Paracelsus has the widest variety of cancer treatments in Europe.

He said, "I don't say we're the best or the most specialized. But we definitely have the largest spectrum. And this enables us to do cancer treatments in an extremely individual way. We treat the person, not the cancer. Our approach to cancer is that there's a cause. Often there's more than one cause.

How Paracelsus cures cancer nature's way

"Strategy One is that we look for the causes, and the more pieces of the puzzle we can find, the better.

"Strategy Two is that we build up the immune system, which is connected to the intestinal milieu. We build that up intensively. Our comprehensive stool analysis reveals food allergies and the extent to which the intestinal flora (beneficial bacteria) have been destroyed. We change nutrition away from the food allergies so the immune system has more strength to fight the cancer. We provide an individualized, correct eating plan for each patient while they're here.

"T-lymph cells [part of the immune system] are located in the small intestine. But they can be paralyzed by a food allergy. It's like what happened to Germany in World War II. The Germans had most of their soldiers on the Eastern Front in Russia, and the Americans came in on the other Front and won the war. Take away the allergen, and the T-lymph cells are released to work on the cancer front."

It certainly makes sense that an eating plan that avoids food allergies frees up the immune system to vanquish the cancer.

Strategy Three is detoxification, which Dr. Rau said is absolutely essential to cure cancer. At Paracelsus, cancer patients usually get two sessions of colonic hydrotherapy each week. Paracelsus uses a closed system of colonic hydrotherapy. This means that the patient doesn't need to use the toilet after the procedure because water enters the colon through a tube and the waste exits the body through the same tube.

This procedure is controlled by a trained colonic hydrotherapist, who massages the patient's abdomen during this painless, cleansing procedure that lasts about an hour. And the patient can see the waste that has just been removed from the colon pass through the clear plastic tube. The closed system of colonic hydrotherapy is a clean, odorless, efficient way to get rid of the garbage from the intestinal tract. Following this garbage removal, Paracelsus repopulates the gut with the beneficial bacteria needed for good health. This is called reflorestation, which gives the immune system a boost.

Cleansing the colon is only one aspect of detoxification. Getting rid of heavy metals such as mercury is another.

But dental mercury is safe, right? Wrong!

Cancer patients often have a problem with heavy metal toxicity, and Paracelsus uses a variety of therapies to get rid of heavy metals such as mercury. Contrary to what you may have heard from conventional dentists about the "safety" of mercury in dental fillings, it's a problem.

Dr. Rau told us that dental pathologies are the underlying cause of many cancers. That's why each cancer patient at Paracelsus gets a dental examination that includes a panoramic X-ray. This X-ray is evaluated by a physician and a dentist.

In fact, one of the dentists I interviewed at Paracelsus, Frank Pleus, D.D.S., is also a licensed, practicing M.D. and also an oral surgeon!

Dental fillings containing mercury — often known as amalgam or "silver" fillings — need to be removed and replaced with a biologically compatible filling. Replacing amalgam fillings reduces the body's toxic load, but it must be done carefully. Otherwise toxic fumes can be released, leaving the patient with even more mercury poisoning. The biological dentists at Paracelsus are experts at safely removing and replacing toxic fillings.

Root canals and other infections of the jawbone are linked to many cancers, according to Dr. Rau. He said that 147 out of 150 breast cancer patients at Paracelsus had root-canal infected teeth on the meridian that includes the breast. But only 35 percent of non-breast cancer patients had root canals on that meridian.

Every cancer patient at Paracelsus sees one of the biological dentists to determine if any dental problems need to be addressed as part of the individualized cancer treatment plan. The dentists have a sophisticated lab that can manufacture ceramic crowns and bridges on site.

The therapy that gave actor Steve McQueen the upper hand over his cancer

Dr. Rau told me about a therapy Paracelsus offers that's almost impossible to find anywhere else: organ cell extract therapy.

Dr. Rau said, "We're the only clinic in Switzerland — there's another one in Germany — that's allowed to do organ cell extract therapy. We have specific permission from the state to do it because we can prove that the cells are clean. We use live cells from the liver and thymus of newborn animals. We don't kill the animals to get their live cells. Rather, we get the liver and thymus from lambs, calves, and piglets that would be killed anyway for their meat at the butcher shop.

"When these animals go to the slaughterhouse, our veterinarian is there to test and verify that the animals are clean. The animals come from free-ranging herds that have been grass-fed for generations. The animals are totally organic. After taking the liver and thymus, we make a preparation out of the healthy, fresh, juvenile cells. You have to break down the cell wall through the osmotic process to get to the inner part, which has healing substances."

It's rare to find a cancer clinic that offers organ cell extract therapy. I first heard about this therapy when I interviewed the last surviving doctor from the medical team that treated movie star Steve McQueen for his mesothelioma in Mexico. McQueen's medical team, which included a doctor flown in from Germany, gave him organ cell extract therapy, and he was actually beating his cancer. McQueen died not from cancer but from a low potassium level and from complications of an elective surgery.

A wide range of therapies

Cancer patients who come to Paracelsus undergo a wide variety of immune-boosting, detoxifying, and anti-cancer therapies over a three week period. During that time, the patient's white blood cells renew themselves totally, according to Dr. Rau.

Dr. Rau said that some patients ask what can be done in addition to chemo and radiation while other patients only want biological (natural) treatment. "I like the second group better," said Dr. Rau. That's because he has more confidence in natural treatments. Dr. Rau sometimes administers low-dose chemo but only when it's absolutely necessary. Because the chemo is low-dose, his patients who receive chemo experience no side effects: no nausea, no vomiting, no hair-loss.

Almost all cancer patients need intensive detoxification, especially those who've had high-dose chemo from a conventional cancer doctor.

Paracelsus empowers patients to take charge of their health

Dr. Rau said, "We once asked our patients what's the most important thing we provided. They said it was that we gave them the means of curing themselves, that we taught them how to integrate themselves into the treatment: how to change their eating plan, their attitude, their thinking."

This answer surprised the Paracelsus doctors. They had expected the patients to say that the treatments were the most important thing.

In Dr. Rau's opinion, "Any cancer doctor who says none of his patients die is a liar. I couldn't say that 90 percent profit from our treatment, but at least 70 to 80 percent get a better quality of life. And many get a much longer lifespan than they were told."

Sadly, many cancer patients wait until they're at Stage Four, then decide to go to Paracelsus as a last resort. When cancer patients reach Stage Four, conventional cancer doctors typically tell them to put their affairs in order because they have just a few months or weeks to live.

Of course, it would be better not to wait until Stage Four to seek alternative treatment. But the doctors at Paracelsus have impressive success stories even with these late-stage patients.

"Hopeless" cancer patient from Brazil beats her cancer

For example, Dr. Rau accepted one such "hopeless" cancer patient from Brazil. "Maria" (not her real name) was about 60 years old when Dr. Rau first saw her. She had ovarian cancer with metastasis to the liver.

Maria had had surgery, chemo, and radiation — all that conventional cancer medicine could offer her — but to no avail. When she came to the clinic, she looked terrible. Her whole abdomen was jam-packed with cancer, and she had such a buildup of fluid in her abdomen that she looked like she was nine months pregnant.

Dr. Rau said his colleagues were shocked that he would admit a patient who had so little hope. "Are you crazy?," they privately asked him. "She's half dead! She'll die!"

But Maria was at Paracelsus, and Dr. Rau felt an obligation to do his best for her. He gave her mistletoe and high-dose ozone directly into the abdominal space, and every other day he gave her low-dose chemo. When Maria left the clinic after six weeks of treatment, she looked good. The excess fluid was all gone.

Six months later Dr. Rau called Maria to see how she was doing. She told him she was busy doing her housework. She said she had no more pain, no more bloating, and a good quality of life. Though it was too early to tell if she was cured for good, no one could deny that Paracelsus changed her life.

Lactic acid therapy: fighting fire with fire

One of the most unusual cancer treatments Paracelsus offers is lactic acid therapy, which neutralizes the lactic acid that enables cancer to hide from the immune system.

Here's how that therapy works. Unlike normal cells, cancer cells create their energy based on glucose fermentation. This anaerobic fermentation produces lactic acid. The lactic acid that surrounds the cancer allows the cancer to hide from the immune system.

Dr. Rau said, "How do we neutralize lactic acid? Right-spin lactic acid neutralizes the cancer cells' left-spin lactic acid, making a neutral molecule. It's a chemical expression."

Dr. Rau used this therapy on a breast cancer patient who had a big tumor infiltrating the muscle. Surgery wasn't an option. So Dr. Rau injected lactic acid directly into and around the cancer. He also injected mistletoe extract and low-dose chemotherapy (about one-twentieth the normal dose). The tumor shrank and shrank until it was completely gone. The patient's conventional doctors couldn't believe the tumor was gone.

Dr. Rau asked me to emphasize that local injections of lactic acid, mistletoe, homeopathic chemotherapy, and ozone into and around cancer tissue are an important form of treatment. He told me, "This treatment is probably one of the most specific and also most locally effective. For example, breast cancer tissue really 'melts' away."

I asked Dr. Rau what he would say to cancer patients who want to use do-it-yourself treatments at home instead of going to a clinic. He said these patients should at least go to a clinic for diagnostics, and then use do-it-yourself treatments at home. He said, "It doesn't matter whether you come here for two weeks or three weeks. You still have to continue doing the program when you return home."

I also sat down for an interview with Dr. Frank Pleus, M.D., D.D.S., O.M.F.S.

Like the other physicians at Paracelsus, Dr. Pleus is an anthroposophical doctor, that is, his practice of medicine is deeply influenced by the theories and discoveries of medical pioneer Dr. Rudolf Steiner.

The profound influence of Rudolf Steiner, the founder of anthroposophical medicine

It was Steiner who first proposed mistletoe treatment for cancer about a hundred years ago. Mistletoe is now a standard treatment for cancer at all of the cancer clinics I visited in Germany, Austria, and Switzerland. It's well established in medical literature that mistletoe has a powerful, direct anti-cancer effect. It also boosts the immune system.

Another aspect of anthroposophical medicine that Paracelsus uses is therapeutic eurhythmy — cardio-sonic treatment — which is a way of teaching patients how to influence their heart rate, manage stress, and relax. Staff therapist Michael Falkner measures the patient's heart rate and breathing with a computer, which generates music. As Dr. Pleus explained, "We call it 'heart-sound' (herz-klang)."

This computer-generated "heart-sound" together with breathing exercises reactivates the parasympathetic nervous system, which Dr. Pleus says is totally suppressed in almost every cancer patient. The parasympathetic and sympathetic nervous systems need to be in proper balance for good health.

As you may know, the sympathetic nervous system is the "fight or flight" part of your nervous system — the part that makes you feel stress. By contrast, the parasympathetic nervous system is the "rest and digest" part — the part that regulates your natural processes like digestion and makes you feel relaxed.

Here's another way to look at it. Your sympathetic nervous system is the accelerator, and your parasympathetic nervous system is the brake. As in driving a car, so it is in life: you need both the accelerator and the brake, which complement each other. But in most cancer patients, the brake is out, and the accelerator is stuck to the floor!

Therapeutic eurhythmy or counseling can fix that problem. It teaches cancer patients how to slow down, manage their stress, and relax so they can heal. This is crucial because stress-run-loose will rip the immune system to shreds.

The therapeutic eurhythmatist Michael Falkner is also the staff psychological counselor. It has been statistically proven that counseling benefits cancer patients.

Dr. Pleus emphasized that cancer patients need to change their lives: "They need to change their stress levels. They need to reactivate their parasympathetic nervous system. They need to re-think what they eat. It's necessary to take self-responsibility. We give the patient an individualized protocol they can follow at home."

Dr. Pleus told me about a Stage Four cancer patient, 70-year-old Barbara from Massachusetts, who had cancer in both of her lungs. Her American doctor told her she had only six months to live. But she didn't accept that death sentence. Instead, she went to Paracelsus.

After getting rid of her cancer at Paracelsus, she returned to Massachusetts to follow the program at home. For exercise, she swims regularly and walks three miles a day. She even visited the ruins of Machu Picchu in the high Andes of Peru.

At the time this is being written, it's too early to know whether Barbara will become a long-term survivor. But a year after she left Paracelsus, Dr. Pleus could say, "She's doing very well."

Dr. Rau's partnership with a German clinic

I also interviewed Dr. Rau's right-hand-man, Dr. Ralf Oettmeier, M.D., who had come to Paracelsus from Klinik im Leben in Greiz, Germany. There's no economic link between the two clinics, but they have a close friendship and an informal partnership.

Because Paracelsus was undergoing some remodeling during my visit, I could hear some construction noise in the background. Dr. Oettmeier remarked, "You can hear our dentist." I laughed.

Dr. Oettmeier told me that Paracelsus doesn't just treat cancer patients but also patients coping with other diseases such as fibromyalgia, Lyme disease, chronic fatigue syndrome, autoimmune diseases, and chronic inflammation. Paracelsus uses hyperthermia for most of these diseases, and all kinds of hyperthermia are available, including transurethral hyperthermia for prostate cancer.

Dr. Oettmeier demonstrated the clinic's sophisticated new darkfield microscope, which is connected to an HD camera system that's connected in real-time to a high resolution screen. He demonstrated this system by taking a sample of my blood and looking at it on the high resolution screen at a magnification of 2,500.

It's amazing to see living blood cells floating across the screen. This diagnostic tool helps motivate the cancer patients to appreciate the wonder of life, and it also gives them encouragement that the treatment is working. When they arrive at the clinic, their blood may not look good under high magnification. But after a week or two of treatment, the patient typically sees a dramatic difference. Dr. Oettmeier tells patients, "This is your movie. These are your living cells. You're going to help them work much better!"

Paracelsus has a daughter clinic in the Italian Alps

During my visit I learned that Paracelsus has a daughter clinic in the Italian Alps. I didn't have time to visit that clinic, but it offers practically all of the therapies the Swiss Paracelsus clinic offers.

One advantage of the Italian clinic is that the hotel rooms are located in the clinic. One disadvantage is that the Italian clinic has no biological dentistry department, but that would only be a disadvantage for those cancer patients who need dental work.

The main clinic near St. Gallen, the one I visited, owns its own small hotel nearby called Hotel Säntis, where the patients get a healthy cancer diet and can do some additional treatments in the evenings, including pulsed magnetic fields, local hyperthermia, and sauna.

How to become a patient at Paracelsus

Paracelsus offers a variety of medical services, including health tune-ups and detoxification. But most patients go to Paracelsus because they have cancer or another degenerative disease.

To be treated at Paracelsus, patients must give a down payment when they arrive. Every week they get a statement listing the services rendered and their current account balance. Then they make another deposit for their second week to cover anticipated services.

The costs vary greatly depending on what kind of medication is recommended and how much dental work is needed. Dental work at Paracelsus Clinic can be expensive, but the clinic has a reputation for doing it right.

If no dental work or expensive medications are needed, treatment at Paracelsus costs about 7,000 Swiss francs the first week and about 4,500 Swiss francs the following weeks, if intensive treatments are needed. The initial costs are rather high because Paracelsus Clinic doctors first do extensive toxicological, cellular, and alternative evaluations before designing an individualized treatment plan.

Because Paracelsus is an outpatient clinic only, it provides no overnight beds. The clinic can advise you about hotel options. Hotel and food costs are not included in the cost for treatments. To get to the clinic you would fly into the nearby Zurich international airport.

Contact information for the main Paracelsus clinic:

Paracelsus Klinik Lustmühle AG

P.O. Box 162 9053 Teufen/AR Switzerland

Head physician: Dr. Thomas Rau, M.D.

Websites: www.drrausway.com
www.paracelsus.ch

e-mail: info@paracelsus.ch

Phone: +41 71 335 71 71

Fax: +41 71 335 71 00

Contact information for the daughter clinic in the Italian Alps:

Paracelsus Clinica Al Ronc

Strada Cantonale 158
CH-6540 Castaneda GR

Website: www.alronc.ch

e-mail: info@alronc.ch

Phone: +41 91 820 40 40

Fax: +41 91 820 40 41

Chapter Ten

Dr. Frank Daudert's clinics in Germany and Austria

The charming town of Bad Aibling, on the edge of the Bavarian Alps, is certainly a good place for Dr. Frank Daudert's Praxisklinik for outpatients. Dr. Daudert divides his time between that clinic and his ProLife clinic in Igls, a tiny village above Innsbruck, Austria. The two clinics are about an hour apart by car.

I interviewed the founder and chief physician, Dr. Frank Daudert, at the ProLife clinic. He told me a remarkable story about a visit in 2003 from a salesman representing one of the best-known drug companies.

The sales rep pulled open his laptop computer and asked Dr. Daudert, "How many patients do you have?" After entering the information into his laptop, he gave Dr. Daudert a business proposition: "O.K. If you give every patient a high dose of chemotherapy, after one year you'll get 3.7 million euros back."

Obviously, the drug company was willing to sneak this 3.7 million euros to Dr. Daudert under the table – with no taxes or reporting.

Without hesitation, Dr. Daudert replied, "I don't need your money."

Drug salesman tells Dr. Daudert, "You're from a different planet"

The sales rep shook his head in disbelief, saying, "Every hospital works together with us. You're from a different planet." As he was walking down the street back to his car he was still shaking his head in disbelief.

To Dr. Daudert it was an easy decision to make. He doesn't give high doses of chemotherapy because that would harm his patients. It would violate the most basic rule of medicine, the ancient motto that says, "First do no harm." High dose chemotherapy is dangerous: it poisons and sometimes kills patients.

Dr. Daudert told me, "Now I understand why so many doctors give high dose chemotherapy." It was crystal clear to me, too.

He says the drug company doesn't like his use of "microchemotherapy" – the low-dose approach – because their sales to his clinic are 80 to 90 percent less than they could be.

Dr. Daudert also told me that researchers brazenly falsify many "scientific" studies that put drugs in a positive light. He knows of one such researcher who made 43 falsifications in his studies. He said, "He isn't in prison, but he should be."

Dr. Daudert made this observation regarding conventional cancer treatment: "Doctors give chemo, chemo, chemo. And patients die, die, die. I only give patients treatments that I would take myself. This is important to understand. Many oncologists who prescribe high-dose chemotherapy refuse to take it when they get cancer."

When Dr. Daudert administers low-dose chemotherapy in conjunction with hyperthermia, it causes no side effects. Patients don't lose their hair. They feel normal. They can go outside and enjoy the fresh air and the charm of Bavaria or Austria. They don't feel sickened, nauseated, and weakened. And he only uses low-dose chemo if testing shows it would help the patient get rid of cancer.

Saving a 55-year-old brain cancer victim from the brink of death

Edith, a 55-year-old woman from the nearby principality of Liechtenstein, came to the clinic with her husband. She had a large brain tumor. She was vomiting and couldn't eat. She needed help in the bathroom. She had balance problems and had difficulty walking. She was suffering seizures. And she wasn't in her right mind, having lost her sense of time.

Edith's doctor in Switzerland had been giving her radiation and high doses of chemotherapy. But these highly toxic therapies had no effect whatsoever on her tumor, which kept growing. In desperation, Edith's husband, a helicopter pilot, drove her to Dr. Daudert's clinic.

Dr. Daudert told me that after just one week of treatment, Edith was eating and walking without difficulty. "The tumor has shrunk by 50 percent. I'll show you pictures," he said.

To shrink this tumor, Dr. Daudert used a variety of therapies combining natural medicine and conventional medicine, including immune-system building and hyperthermia.

Probably everybody produces cancer cells, but...

According to Dr. Daudert, every day a normal healthy body might develop about 100 cancer cells. . .

"But your immune system destroys them. It's a good system. If your body has a weak immune system, cancer cells develop a protein coating the killer cells can't see, and they also build an acid wall to hide behind. We destroy the acid wall with high-dose alkaline infusions. And we destroy the cancer cell's protein wall with special enzymes.

"Food is very important. If the patient eats a lot of sugar, the cancer cells are happy. Without sugar, they're unhappy. Eating the right foods can help patients go from metastasized cancer to a state of health.

"We teach about food, what the patient is supposed to eat. We also have relaxation therapy and psychological counseling. We want the patient to know everything about the disease and how to combat it, and everything about the healing process.

How conventional doctors brainwash patients into dying early

One young man came to the clinic with pancreatic cancer in the early stage, and Dr. Daudert was confident he could cure his cancer. But the patient's doctor had told him, "Studies show that with a pancreatic tumor you have seven months to live." Despite Dr. Daudert's efforts to unbrainwash him and deprogram his negative thinking, this man's wife said, "Every day my husband remembered the oncologist saying 'you have seven months at most.'" He kept on repeating that over and over in his mind. He died exactly on the date that the doctor had predicted.

Dr. Daudert told me, "We instruct the patient to think about healing, not about death. When doctors tell cancer patients, 'You're going to die in three months,' they often die within three months – not because of the cancer but because of the negative prediction: if they believe the doctor, they program themselves to die in three months!

"When a patient first comes to the clinic, our first step is to sit down with the patient for an hour or two and destroy this negative programming and give them new programming. If patients think only of dying, *it's impossible to help them.* As the Bible says, 'If you give up when trouble comes, it shows that you have very little strength' (Proverbs 24:10).

"Five years ago when a doctor told one of our patients 'you'll die in a few months,' she got depressed at first, but then she went back to her doctor and said, 'I've decided to live.' She came to our clinic and is still alive today.

"It's important to discuss the patient's family life and job. Sometimes it's necessary to tell the patient to change their work if it's too stressful. Unmanaged stress depresses the immune system."

Dr. Daudert also explained that there's a link between parasites and cancer. If someone has too many parasites, the immune system can become overextended and unable to deal with cancer cells or bacteria or viruses. Boosting the immune system helps deal with these health problems.

As I walked through the ProLife clinic, it was difficult to keep my attention on it. I couldn't help looking out the windows at the beautiful, incredible alpine views.

Dr. Daudert explained that when some cancer patients first come to the clinic they can hardly move. Some of them say, "My doctor said I can't do anything."

Wrong! Dr. Daudert tells them, "You *must* move." Patients are happier when they're moving, he explains, and their muscles develop with the exercise, too.

Study proves magnetic-field therapy boosts immune system, increases natural killer cells 20 to 25 percent!

As with almost all of the German cancer clinics I visited, one of the key therapies at Dr. Daudert's clinic is magnetic-field therapy. Dr. Daudert explained that this low-energy, low-frequency device comes from Russian space medicine. As the cosmonauts stayed in space for long periods, they encountered health problems. Being away from the earth's magnetic field impaired the function of their organs.

So Russian scientists developed a magnetic-field device the cosmonauts could use in space. The scientists found that cosmonauts needed to use it three times a day to keep their health on an even keel. With magnetic-field therapy, cosmonauts were able to stay in space for a

year and even longer with no problem. NASA also uses magnetic-field therapy to keep U.S. astronauts healthy.

At Dr. Daudert's clinic, the patients get magnetic-field therapy by relaxing on a special mat for 16 minutes, once each day. This therapy supports every organ system in the body and boosts the immune system. It's proven. Dr. Daudert told me, "Two years ago we did a study. We took blood samples from 200 patients on the first day. One hundred patients took magnetic-field therapy, and the other 100 didn't. Patients who took the magnetic-field therapy were found to have 20 to 25 percent MORE immune cells, natural killer cells – the cells that can destroy cancer cells."

No wonder the German cancer clinics use this space-age technology as a key part of the treatment plan.

Laser blood therapy helps astronauts and cancer patients

Dr. Daudert told me about another therapy astronauts need to stay healthy in space: laser blood therapy. This therapy is necessary for astronauts in space to keep up their energy. Dr. Daudert uses this same therapy to benefit his cancer patients.

Here's how it works: A catheter is installed in the vein of the arm. Through the catheter, a laser beam reaches the blood. A short time later, the patient typically says something like this:"I feel good. I can't explain it, but I feel better. I have more energy."

Dr. Daudert said, "Our philosophy is, 'If it's helping, it's good.' It works. Patients with wounds that don't heal can benefit from this therapy. A lady who had an operation for colon cancer had a wound that wouldn't heal. After she had the laser therapy, you could see from day to day that the wound was healing. After just one laser treatment, a man who had not been able to stand up from a sitting position for two years stood up unconsciously. His wife said, 'Hey, you have an appointment.' Standing up, he said,

'An appointment?' And then he realized, with astonishment, that he was standing up."

Dr. Daudert knows, from reviewing "before" and "after" photos, that laser blood therapy boosts the immune cells. He says, "I love space medicine!"

Another doctor at ProLife gave me this explanation for why laser blood therapy works so well: "Usually the red blood cells, which are responsible for energy and oxygen supply, are ellipsoid, and they cannot pass through vessels that are narrower than the diameter of the red blood cells. The laser beam directly improves the malleability of the red blood cells, enabling them to pass through even very small vessels and supply bigger areas with oxygen and energy. The laser beam is also able to activate some immune cells directly."

One therapy at the ProLife clinic that I didn't see at any of the other clinics is a device – a bed – that vibrates the patient not just up and down but also in a three-dimensional way. Dr. Daudert said this device promotes detoxification of poisons, including heavy metals. It cleanses the lymphatic system and benefits the liver and kidneys, too.

During the tour I bumped into the delightful couple from Liechtenstein I told you about earlier: Edith and her husband, the helicopter pilot.

Husband calls wife's recovery from inoperable, terminal brain cancer "Incredible! Unbelievable!"

With unbridled enthusiasm, the husband told us, "I can tell you Edith's brain tumor declined by 50 percent – and that's in just three-and-a-half weeks! Incredible! Incredible! Unbelievable! Our doctors in Switzerland would hardly believe it. They asked me, 'What have you done?' I told them, but they said, 'We don't want to discuss this.' And that's a shame. You can see the X-ray pictures. Incredible."

With my own eyes, I saw Edith walking unassisted with no problems whatsoever. And as far as I could tell, she seemed to be in her right mind. Her husband couldn't have been happier with her recovery.

As a token of international friendship, the husband picked up some treats at a local shop and gave them to me. I accepted this thoughtful gift with pleasure.

Dr. Daudert said he's had many successes with patients such as Edith who've come to his clinic with inoperable brain tumors. He's even had success with the deadliest form of brain cancer, glioblastoma multiforme. A 40-year-old German patient came to Dr. Daudert's clinic with stage-four "glio" – as it's called for short. At the time I spoke with Dr. Daudert, the patient was 45 years old and doing fine.

Dr. Daudert has an insatiable appetite for discovering what works in medicine. He has traveled the world, seeking out "medicine men" to learn about their natural medicines.

How a Siberian medicine man cures cancer with snake venom!

Dr. Daudert told me an amazing story about a medicine man he met in an isolated corner of the Siberian wilderness. This area is so remote there's no physician within a 250-mile radius, so the villagers all depended on the medicine man for their health. A woman came to him with a large, ugly tumor of the breast. He let Dr. Daudert examine his patient. The cancer was obviously severe.

The woman had no money to take the train to Moscow for treatment in a cancer clinic there. She had only the medicine man to help her. She put her life in his hands.

The medicine man told her, "No problem." And then he left.

His wife told Dr. Daudert, "He's looking for a snake. He needs the venom."

He came back with a poisonous snake, from which he milked the venom. Then he mixed the fresh venom with raw honey and covered the tumor with a poultice made from the venom/honey mixture. Just three days later the tumor had shrunk by 20 percent! The woman was happy. Her pain was gone!

Doctors at the University of Moscow heard about the effectiveness of the medicine man's cancer cure and are now studying snake venom for its medicinal value. While other Russian industries have their share of problems, Dr. Daudert explains that there's no "pharmaceutical mafia" in Russia to hamper, discourage, or discredit such research into natural medicines.

Dr. Daudert runs tests that show that no chemotherapy whatsoever will be helpful for some patients. He says, "Doctors are blindly giving chemotherapy to some patients while the cancer cells smile and the patients die."

Colonic hydrotherapy is "very important" for cancer patients

According to Dr. Daudert, colonic hydrotherapy is "very important." Indeed, all the German physicians I interviewed agreed foursquare on the importance of colonic hydrotherapy. A gunked-up gut goes with disease, but a clean, efficiently functioning gut goes with health.

Dr. Daudert says colonic hydrotherapy is so important that he teaches the patients how to do it at home and keep up their colonics.

Another important tool at the clinic is the darkfield microscope – the device I've mentioned before that magnifies the patient's living blood 14,000 times. This microscope enables a trained doctor to see what's really going on with the patient's health.

You can find more information about how doctors use the darkfield microscope in cancer treatment in one of my other books, *America's Best Cancer Doctors and Their Secrets*, which is available on my publisher's website, www.CancerDefeated.com.

The heart of ProLife is the biological kitchen, which only uses fruits and vegetables from organic sources. Dr. Daudert told us, "The food is *really* organic. We know the farmers. This is very important."

Dr. Daudert said, "My wife Angelica works side by side with me in this clinic. I'm very happy. She works too much. When I call the clinic from Bad Aibling at 10:00 p.m., she's still at the clinic. I tell her, 'You must go home.'"

Dr. Daudert is the head of the ProLife clinic, but Angelica is its heart. She does much more than manage the clinic so it runs like clockwork, a demanding task that requires meticulous attention to detail. She knows the patients and lovingly helps care for them. Her husband said, "She's the mother of the house. She's great."

Mrs. Daudert's extraordinary compassion for the patients

Two weeks earlier, when twin sisters were staying at the clinic, the healthy twin became totally exhausted from sleeping in the same room with her gravely ill sister. Angelica said she would take her place and sleep with the ill sister for a night so the other twin could relax for a night.

When would anything like that ever happen in an American hospital?

"Patients must feel the positive energy from doctors, nurses, everyone on the staff," Dr. Daudert told us. "Everyone on our staff is part of the team. We have six doctors, plus nurses and physical therapists. If a doctor notices that a patient is depressed, we give special attention to pull the patient out of it."

Here's how Dr. Daudert described what the cancer patients experience at ProLife:

"Most people stay two to four weeks. The first appointment with the doctor takes a long time because it's necessary to go through the patient's history. We take the patient's blood, analyze it in the lab, and get the results. We create a treatment plan that includes such things as hyperthermia, magnetic-field therapy, colonics, injections, Chinese medicine, and so on."

Dr. Daudert paid a heavy price in the struggle for freedom

When Dr. Daudert was growing up on the Eastern side of the Iron Curtain, he didn't understand why there was a Berlin Wall. His parents weren't Communists, and he belonged to a pro-freedom group in his church. Being part of such a group was dangerous in those days.

In 1982 the Communists infiltrated his church to see who was involved in the freedom movement. The secret police identified him as one of the ringleaders and began spying on him and following him.

Three years later, when he was 24, the Communists arrested and imprisoned him for promoting freedom. He didn't understand why he was behind bars. He'd done nothing wrong.

He knew he needed a Bible, but that seemed like an impossible dream. How can you get a Bible behind bars in a Communist prison? When he asked his atheistic guards for a Bible, they just sneered. But he kept on asking. About a week later, amazingly, one of the guards threw a Bible at him.

Other prisoners asked, "You have a Bible? How did you get it?" He told them, "You have to ask for one."

Though at first he didn't understand why he was behind bars, he soon realized he was there to help other people in the prison. Many, having been raised under atheistic Communism, knew absolutely nothing about God or the Bible. And the idealistic, good-hearted 24-year-old Frank Daudert felt called to teach them.

Dr. Daudert told us, "The Word of God is the biggest power we have. When I had a Bible in prison, I felt the power. I read for other prisoners who had never heard about the Bible." The Communists kept him behind bars for one year – an experience that left an indelible imprint on him. Perhaps it was the year he spent in a Communist prison that gave him the strength of character to refuse any bribe, no matter how lucrative.

At ProLife I also interviewed Dr. Adem Günes, M.D., an energetic young medical researcher who had done a major research project there. When he told me about his work, I was truly astonished.

Conventional cancer doctors doubt the effectiveness of complementary treatments. They claim, "You don't have studies. You can't prove what you say." Dr. Günes embarked on a research project to prove them dead wrong. When I interviewed him, he was near the end of the project. His goal is to make complementary oncology more accepted by conventional doctors.

Dr. Günes chose the top 20 cancers and researched what's known about those cancers. He collected studies from around the world to analyze which herbal or complementary therapies work and which ones don't. He read roughly 1,500 studies on lung cancer alone. Based on that research, he has identified the herbal substances that are definitely effective against lung cancer. He has tested these substances on cancer cells in the clinic's lab and found that indeed they killed the cancer cells. One of these substances, artemesia, is particularly effective against lung cancer.

Dr. Günes told me, "No one can say that hyperthermia is unproved and untested. It should be more accepted. Here at the clinic we have the world's biggest database on herbal and complementary substances – over 100,000 studies. There aren't more studies than this. We've read and studied and analyzed every study! It was hard work. Two secretaries supported the research. It's a golden treasure. We're testing substance after substance to see what works and what doesn't work in vitro [in a lab culture]."

This discovery made the hair on Dr. Günes's arm stand up!

Dr. Günes told me, "There are 50,000 substances in our database. We've found one substance that's particularly effective on cancer such as colon, melanoma, prostate, and monocarcinoma. We were shocked. I talked to a biologist and another scientist from a university hospital, and they had never seen anything more effective at killing cancer cells while leaving healthy cells undisturbed. It's not chemo. It's an herb that destroys cancer cells by inducing apoptosis. The next step will be to test it in vivo [on a living organism]."

How does the substance work? As Dr. Günes explained, "Apoptosis is programmed cell death. It's one of the most effective methods to stop uncontrolled multiplication. Tumor cells have lost this ability. They multiply and multiply and multiply, causing tumors to grow. The substance activates a special enzyme to activate apoptosis in cancer cells. The substance has no effect on healthy cells. **Even my hairs are standing every time when I discuss this stuff.**"

Dr. Günes had me on the edge of my chair. He said the plant from which the substance comes is well known in Asia and the Middle East. It has a long history as a remedy for just about every ailment, according to literature a few hundred years old. The name of the substance is black cumin, but it's also known as black caraway, black sesame, onion seed, and Roman coriander. Its official name is *Nigella sativa*, and it's often called "black seed."

Black cumin is so powerful it could replace chemo!

Dr. Günes said, "I'm convinced it will work well in vivo. I told my scientists, 'Repeat every test five times, not just three times.' When we started, we told our scientists to find substances that could enhance the chemo effect. After we found such substances, the scientists said, 'We don't need enhancement for chemo. We've found an *alternative* to chemo!' This was new. It wasn't even our goal in the beginning! We couldn't have imagined that there are so many substances that could be so effective."

Regarding the top 20 cancers, I asked Dr. Günes whether he has identified the substances that work for each of these cancers. He replied yes. I asked if there's much difference in the protocol to use for each type of cancer. He said, "Yes. A huge difference!"

Black cumin and some of the other effective natural substances haven't yet been tested on humans because Dr. Günes said it isn't possible to have clinical trials with human patients. But he observed that some cancer patients don't have a lot of time, and he said, "With little time available, we may be able to use these substances on terminal patients."

100% success rate for the deadliest brain cancer!

Dr. Günes said, "The next step will be to combine herbal therapies. We're now more successful. With the last four brain cancer patients, we have a 100 percent success rate. These brain cancers were glioblastoma multiforme. It grows quickly. It needs lots of blood vessels to grow, and we found a way to stop the vessels from growing. That's why we were so successful."

One of the four most recent brain cancer patients is a German who was given a runaround by his medical insurance company. His first request for insurance coverage was denied. After Dr. Daudert's treatments shrank the tumor, he appealed the denial. The insurance company said, "We need a report from your neurologist." The neurologist compared the "before" and "after" MRIs and had to admit the tumor was smaller, but he said, "I don't think it's because of the therapy at Dr. Daudert's clinic." So the insurance company denied his request again. After he could document even more improvement, he appealed a third time. The neurologist told the insurance company, "The tumor is smaller, and I don't know why." The insurance company finally agreed to pay for the treatment.

Ted Kennedy's disease
can be beaten!

Glioblastoma multiforme is considered the deadliest kind of brain cancer. It's the kind that killed Ted Kennedy. Even Kennedy's multimillion dollar fortune couldn't buy him a cure from America's top conventional cancer doctors. It's astonishing that Dr. Daudert was able to cure four out of four of his most recent cases of glioblastoma multiforme brain cancer.

Like some of the top cancer clinics in Germany, Dr. Daudert prescribes Thalidomide to shut off the blood supply to the brain tumor. When used correctly, this drug is apparently safe for adults. The only side effect is sleepiness. But women who are pregnant or who may become pregnant must not take it because it would impede the normal development of the child in the womb!

How to determine
the best therapies

Dr. Daudert said his clinic has made a vast improvement in its diagnostics. He can do a genetic analysis from circulating tumor cells. He can isolate the circulating tumor cells in the blood to analyze their structure and determine what will be effective in killing the tumor cell.

Dr. Günes said that in all of Europe he knows of only three clinics that do such a test. Dr. Daudert's clinic is one of them. It's complicated and expensive to do this test, but it's worth it to help the patient avoid unnecessary chemo and to find the most effective therapies. It's not like a well-known Greek blood test that has the same aim. It's a more specific test, Dr. Günes said.

As Dr. Günes explained, even if cancer patients get rid of the tumor, they almost certainly still have tumor cells circulating in their blood. The *only* answer is to improve the immune system so that it mops up the remaining tumor cells. Otherwise, the cancer will come back. To boost the immune system, the clinic uses a product from Japan that contains a substance from rice hulls in combination with the shiitake mushroom.

A few months after my visit, Dr. Günes left ProLife to become an independent medical consultant.

Dr. Daudert's nutritional
recommendations

Dr. Daudert told me that his clinic now recommends the Budwig protocol in combination with the low carb aspects of the Coy diet. For patients who have a sweet tooth, he recommends a sugar substitute that doesn't feed cancer. The name of the product is "Naturally Sweet." It's a natural sugar from a melon, but the human body can't use it, Dr. Daudert explained. I sampled a piece of cake that uses this alternative to sugar, and it certainly tasted like a real dessert.

Every patient gets personal instruction on how to eat well so they can stay healthy when they return home. This instruction, which lasts at least an hour, is crucial because Dr. Daudert believes you can keep cancer away by eating correctly. That's a better alternative than digging your own grave with your teeth.

The government won't allow Dr. Daudert to use whole-body hyperthermia at his ProLife clinic in Austria, but he's freely able to use it in his clinic in Bad Aibling on the German side of the border. Dr. Daudert believes that moderate "long term" whole-body hyperthermia for eight hours is more effective than extreme hyperthermia for two hours. He's seeing good results with this approach.

Here are some stories that demonstrate what Dr. Daudert's clinics can accomplish.

16-year-old girl narrowly avoids amputation!

Dr. Daudert told me about a 16-year-old girl from Vienna with bone cancer on her shoulder. Her doctors in Vienna said, "We have to amputate your arm, or you'll die." Her father said no, and looked for an alternative. He brought her to Dr. Daudert's clinic, where she got local hyperthermia and herbs.

This therapy shrank the tumor quickly, enabling the doctors in Vienna to remove it surgically without amputating the arm. They were impressed with the results, but they didn't call Dr. Daudert to ask "what did you do" or "how did you shrink that tumor so quickly." They didn't seem interested.

Even though the surgery was successful, the oncologist in Vienna told the father, "She needs chemo or she won't see Christmas!" This death prediction frightened the father. He didn't want to lose his precious daughter. In a panic, he called Dr. Daudert for advice. But instead of bringing his daughter back to him, the father knuckled under to the other doctor's bullying, and put her on chemo. Dr. Daudert said, "We never saw this patient again. We have no idea whether she's alive or dead."

For the third time, what's your name?

A 55-year-old man from Frankfurt baffled his doctors while keeping a *huge* secret from them. Conventional cancer doctors in Frankfurt treated him for a big tumor on his leg. They gave him industrial-strength chemo and radiation, which had no effect on the tumor. His doctors had nothing more to offer, so he went to Dr. Daudert's clinic for hyperthermia, immune-boosting therapies, herbal therapies, and detoxification. These therapies healed him completely!

Without telling his conventional doctors in Frankfurt where he had been or what he had done, he returned to them after six months for a follow-up examination. The cancer was 100 percent gone. The doctors compared the "before" and "after" PET scans, and what they were looking at didn't make any sense to them. Three times the doctors asked him, "What's your name? What's your date of birth?" They couldn't believe the two pictures were of the same patient!

The Frankfurt doctors wrote in his record, "We are proud that the chemo finally worked after six months." This is laughable. He never did tell his local doctors about his treatments at Dr. Daudert's clinic because he didn't want any problems. Some doctors get so offended that a patient would seek treatment elsewhere, they won't even agree to monitor the patient.

Munich doctor says, "We must amputate your foot"

When a woman from Munich got melanoma of the foot, her local doctor told her, "The cancer is in a difficult area. We have to amputate." The tumor was deep. She was at stage four. Desperate, she went to Dr. Daudert's clinic, looking for a miracle.

Three weeks later her cancer was completely gone, but not because of a miracle. The cancer went away because of sound medical treatment, including hyperthermia, immune-boosting therapies, detoxification, and Galvano therapy. In Galvano therapy, the cancer is "zapped" by a mild, carefully controlled electrical current – just enough to kill the cancer. Galvano therapy is especially effective on breast cancer.

She comes back to the clinic for followup visits every three months for immune-boosting therapies. Dr. Daudert said, "We want to make sure the last cancer cell is killed, and the immune system accomplishes that task."

Opera star lost her lung power

Dr. Daudert told me about an opera star who sang every year at the Wagner festival in Bayreuth, Germany. When her breast cancer spread to her lungs, she no longer had the lung power to sing through a five-hour Wagner opera. At Dr. Daudert's clinic she got hyperthermia, insulin potentiation therapy (IPT), and other therapies. These therapies saved not only her life but her career, enabling her to return to the stage at the legendary Bayreuth *Festspielhaus*.

A father lies to save his daughter's life

A university cancer clinic gave a young lady named Tamara two weeks to live. She was bedridden and had stopped eating because she was in the final stage of breast cancer with metastasis all over. Her father, desperate for a solution, called Dr. Daudert and said, "My daughter has a big problem. Can we come *right now*?"

Dr. Daudert asked, "Can she walk?" He replied yes. "Can she eat?" He replied yes.

So Tamara's father brought her into the Praxisklinik in Bad Aibling. It was immediately obvious that she couldn't walk or eat. Dr. Daudert asked, "Why didn't you tell me she couldn't walk or eat?" He said, "I was worried that if I said that, you'd say you couldn't do anything for her." Dr. Daudert could see that he faced a huge challenge. Tamara was conscious, so he looked into her eyes and said, "Tamara, will you fight?" She had no energy, but she managed to say, "Yes. I will fight." Dr. Daudert said, "Then we'll start today!"

Right then and there he gave Tamara one hour of hyperthermia on her liver and lungs, plus immune-boosting infusions and injections. Tamara started feeling better. Each day she perked up a little more. After three weeks she was back on her feet, but she still had metastasis in her bones and needed more treatments. Tamara is a horse therapist who had worked primarily with children. She was eager to get back to helping children with her horse therapy.

About a week later the mayor of Tamara's village came to see Dr. Daudert to thank him. He said, "It's a miracle! We're so happy to see Tamara!" Dr. Daudert replied that perhaps in three months she could return to horse therapy. The mayor exclaimed, "Three months? She's in the forest right now doing horse therapy!"

Five years later this amazing young horse therapist was still "as healthy as a horse." Her PET scan showed no tumor activity. Her father triumphantly brought the scan to the university cancer doctor who, five years earlier, had given Tamara only two weeks to live. He just shook his head and stubbornly insisted that Dr. Daudert's treatments were "wrong." Astonished at this doctor's refusal to consider the possibility that he was wrong himself, the father told him, "I don't see any good treatments at your clinic."

Tamara's case shows that the immune system can heal even advanced-stage cancer as long as the immune cells can recognize the tumor cells as a target. One special quality of Dr. Daudert is that even when everyone else doubts that the patient can live, he says, "Telling patients they have 'two months' or 'three months' to live is wrong because it depresses them and takes away their power. Doctors must speak in a positive way with the patients. A good outcome is possible. Each patient has a chance! We can't heal the patients. The patients can heal themselves." He's not always sure of a good outcome, but he knows it's always possible. He gets energy from seeing his patients improve.

Young man survives the other deadly brain cancer

It bears repeating that Dr. Daudert has demonstrated success in case after case of glioblastoma brain cancer, curing his last four "glio" patients in a row. Conventional doctors fail miserably with this kind of cancer.

The other deadly brain cancer is astrocytoma; patient survival of more than three years is unheard of. Twenty years ago, one of Dr. Daudert's friends was diagnosed with this disease. Four months after brain surgery the tumor came back. Instead of seeking more conventional treatment, he asked Dr. Daudert to help him.

Dr. Daudert gave him local hyperthermia to the brain – the first time he had ever done this therapy for brain cancer. The treatments, which required special infusions to keep the pressure in the brain under control, neutralized the tumor. This patient should have been dead within three years, according to well established medical experience and statistics. But he lived for 19 years with the astrocytoma tumor. This is unheard of. Dr. Daudert deserves worldwide headlines for his successes with astrocytoma and glioblastoma brain cancers.

Father tells doctors to stop torturing his daughter!

A 15-year-old girl with leukemia had been run through the wringer of conventional cancer treatment by the time she came to Dr. Daudert seeking help. The conventional treatment had failed miserably. Her stomach and skin were swollen. Her skin was damaged. And her pain was unbearable.

When the doctors said they wanted to give her even more chemotherapy, her father put his foot down and said, "You've given her round after round of chemotherapy, which has practically destroyed my daughter, and now your answer is that you want to give her more chemotherapy?" He refused the treatment and took his daughter home to die.

By the time the father took his daughter to the Praxisklinik in Bad Aibling, his daughter had been bedridden for three months, and her immune system and blood-building system were down. Dr. Daudert looked into her eyes and asked a question he asked other patients: "Do you want to fight?" She said yes.

He gave her a gentle therapeutic regimen because she was so weak. He reintroduced

probiotics to her intestinal tract and gave her high-dose vitamin infusions and other infusions against the tumor cells, such as B17 (laetrile) plus an herbal remedy. He also gave her special medicine to support the liver, kidneys, and other systems. She felt a little better each day, and by the fourth day she wanted to go back to school.

The father took her home, but she didn't come back for followup as scheduled. Dr. Daudert assumed she had died. With a heavy heart, Dr. Daudert picked up the phone to offer the father condolences for losing his daughter. But the father said, "I couldn't bring her for the appointment because she wanted to go back to school."

Delighted to hear that news, Dr. Daudert made special arrangements to treat her in the evening so she could keep on attending school. After three months there were no cancer cells or leukemia cells in her blood, and her skin was totally healed. Dr. Daudert told me, "Now she's a young woman. Before Christmas she came here with her father and friends to sing Christmas carols on the street."

Dying mother says, "I have a small boy who needs me"

Fifty-year-old Angelika got bad news when a doctor at a university clinic said her pharyngeal cancer was inoperable. He gave her no hope. She was swollen and in terrible shape. She hadn't eaten properly for a while. When she came to Dr. Daudert's clinic she had a strong reason to live. She said, "I have to get healthy because I have a small boy, and he needs his mother."

Her husband firmly supported her. He asked Dr. Daudert, "Does my wife have a chance?" He replied, "Yes, she has a chance," and immediately gave her 2,000 calories per day through a nutritional IV with protein, fat, and a little sugar. (Normally, nutritional IVs are high in sugar.) He also gave her hyperthermia and other therapies. Seven months later the inoperable tumor had disappeared. Now, five years later, she's still cancer free. Dr. Daudert calls her "Miracle Angelika."

The people in her village are delighted to have her back. They all love and appreciate her. They were so impressed with Angelika's cure that they invited Dr. Daudert to speak to a group of interested villagers about what they can do to boost their immune system and prevent cancer.

Two-pack-a-day smoker beats cancer and still smokes like a chimney

Five years ago Pius, a man from Switzerland, came to the clinic with mesothelioma, a cancer of the lining of the lung that's caused by asbestos inhalation. He'd worked in a factory and regularly inhaled asbestos because he never wore a mask. Now seriously ill, he had trouble breathing. To make matters worse, he also smoked two packs of cigarettes a day.

A doctor at a university cancer clinic told him, "I'm sorry. We have no chemo or radiation for this tumor. We can do nothing. You have months to live." His own family doctor piled on when he said, "I'm sure nobody can help you. No doctor in the world can help you. Take a trip around the world." He replied, "I don't need a trip around the world. I need healing!"

At least his family doctor was educable. After Dr. Daudert had treated Pius for a while, his family doctor saw the results and said, "I don't understand. I've never seen such results for this kind of tumor. Go back to that clinic and continue with their treatments!" Because mesothelioma is such a tough cancer, Pius needed local hyperthermia three hours a day for three weeks. He also got B17 (laetrile), herbal remedies, and immune-boosting medicine. He stubbornly refused to quit his two-pack-a-day cigarette habit.

Four months after he started Dr. Daudert's treatment, Pius's cancer completely disappeared, as proven by a CT scan in Switzerland. Upon viewing the scan, the Swiss doctor couldn't believe his eyes. He remarked, "I don't understand. There's nothing to see." He kept on comparing the X-rays of the tumor taken in 2010 with the CT scan from February of 2011, and he was flabbergasted to see no trace of the tumor.

Then something extraordinary happened. Swiss medical insurance companies don't pay for treatment outside Switzerland. But in Pius's case the results were so spectacular that his Swiss insurance company paid for the treatment as a tip of the hat to Dr. Daudert! The doctor for the insurance company said, "I've never seen such success in the case of mesothelioma."

Pius returns to the clinic each year for followup. One year Dr. Daudert's wife saw him smoking outside the clinic. She approached him and said, "I don't understand you! You're healthy. You haven't died. And you still smoke?" He was offended with her for a whole year. Even though he never smokes in the clinic, he smokes so heavily that his clothes reek of stale cigarette smoke. Whenever he enters the clinic he brings the stench with him. It's hard to believe that Pius, still smoking like a chimney, has passed his five-year cancer survival milestone.

One of Pius's relatives, also from Switzerland, came to Dr. Daudert's clinic for her stomach cancer. When I visited, she was nearing her five-year survival milestone.

Insurance company calls woman's 10-year cancer survival "impossible"

A woman named Gisele, who survived a deadly cancer of the bone marrow, is another "miracle" story of Dr. Daudert. When the insurance company had paid for 10 years of her followup medical treatments, an insurance company official wrote Dr. Daudert a letter saying, "We are no longer going to pay claims for this patient because it is impossible for anyone with this diagnosis to live longer than 10 years. The diagnosis must be mistaken."

Dr. Daudert called the University of Frankfurt and asked for Gisele's biopsy material. The University still had it. Dr. Daudert sent it to a lab for analysis and got a report that it was indeed bone marrow cancer, which had been correctly diagnosed the first time.

Now Gisele has passed her 20-year cancer survival milestone. She's not cured, however. She still has some signs of cancer cells, and Dr. Daudert gives her whole-body hyperthermia and infusions to kill them. She feels good. Her disease is chronic, but she's in a state of stable disease, and her quality of life is excellent. Stable disease is like a stalemate in chess where neither side gains the upper hand. But keeping cancer under control counts as a win for the patient!

Patient feedback about the ProLife Klinik

I sent out an e-mail to everyone who bought the first edition of *German Cancer Breakthrough*, requesting feedback – positive or negative – from customers who actually went to one of the clinics I recommended. One customer gave me feedback about Dr. Daudert.

Allen from Switzerland wrote, "I had two large, ugly tumors on the side of my face. The big Zurich University hospital first wanted to do a huge operation, then radiation. I refused. [Dr. Daudert's clinic] first used local area hyperthermia, which had some major effect, but the tumors started heavy bleeding, so it was discontinued after four days. Then they switched to a biological [herbal] chemo. I can't spell its name. This really made a huge change, and the tumors are rapidly decreasing in size. Dr. Daudert estimated a 70 percent reduction two weeks ago, and they are even smaller now. It cost a lot more than I thought it would, but the fast results outweigh any niggles. Every non-European I met at the clinic was there because of your book."

Dr. Daudert told me, "Your book is very important for telling patients what is possible.

Many don't know anything about biological medicine. We're happy that you give information to patients."

How to get to Dr. Daudert's Praxisklinik

To get to Dr. Daudert's Praxisklinik in Bad Aibling you fly to Munich, and the clinic will send a driver to pick you up at the airport. The clinic is only about an hour's drive from Munich. A big advantage of the Praxisklinik is that it's located in one of Germany's finest spa towns. Bad Aibling's new Therme (spa complex) is just a 10-minute walk from the Praxisklinik. The Therme features an amazing complex of pools and saunas. The Therme also offers therapeutic massage, including a whole-body treatment with Bad Aibling's famous mineral-rich mud.

To get to Dr. Daudert's ProLife Klinik in Igls, Austria, you fly into Innsbruck. The clinic will send a driver to pick you up at the airport. It may be better to choose the Bad Aibling clinic because, at the time of this writing, the government won't allow whole-body hyperthermia at the Igls clinic.

Cost of treatment

The cost of treatment is similar to that of other clinics in Germany. It depends on how long a patient stays at the clinic and what kind of treatments are necessary. Treatment for three weeks costs about as much as a minivan. Before a patient comes to the ProLife Klinik, the doctor can provide a more accurate estimate of costs along with the treatment plan. Patients are encouraged to bring a friend or relative for support.

Because of Dr. Daudert's impressive results and the positive feedback about him, I continue to recommend him.

Contact information for Dr. Daudert's ProLife Klinik in Igls/Innsbruck, Austria:

Pro Leben Klinik

Hilberstraße 3
A – 6080 Igls/Innsbruck, Austria

Contact: Dr. Frank Daudert

Website: www.prolife-center.de

e-mail: contact@prolife-center.de

Phone: 011-43-5123-798-62

Fax: 011-43-5123-798-625

Contact information for Dr. Daudert's outpatient clinic in Bad Aibling, Germany:

Stiftung Pro Leben (Pro Life Foundation)

Praxisklinik

Frühlingstraße 30
D-83043 Bad Aibling

Contact: Dr. Frank Daudert

Website: www.praxis-daudert.com

e-mail: info@praxis-daudert.com

Phone: 011-49-8061-497-80

Fax: 011-49-8061-497-829

Chapter Eleven

Dr. Friedrich Douwes's St. Georg Klinik in Bad Aibling

If cancer may be compared to a dragon, many people from around the world have slain it at Klinik St. Georg. The iconic St. George is normally shown slaying a dragon, and many such icons are displayed at the clinic, which is located just across the street from one of the town's baroque-style Catholic churches.

From now on in this chapter, I'll call the clinic "St. George" because the German spelling ("Georg" – pronounced GAYorg) is unfamiliar to Americans.

Like Bad Mergentheim, Bad Bergzabern, and Bad Salzhausen, the town of Bad Aibling, where this clinic is located, is a spa town. In fact, the town has opened a new Therme (pool and sauna complex), which is stunning. It's easy to go by foot through the local park to the Therme, which is famous for the mud treatments. I went to the Therme and got myself smeared with Bad Aibling mud from head to toe. It was a remarkably relaxing and rejuvenating experience.

But patients at St. George don't have to go to the Therme for a mudpack with Bad Aibling mud. They can get that right at St. George, as well as medical baths and spa treatments such as whole body massages and partial massages.

On the wall in the entryway of St. George I noticed a world map with pins stuck all over. Each pin signified that a patient had come to St. George from that country or region. The countries and regions include Siberia, Canada, the United States, Central America, South America, England, Spain, Belgium, Sweden, Russia, Kazakhstan, Iran, Arabia, Yemen, Tanzania, Indonesia, and Australia.

When I first arrived at St. George, Dr. Douwes was ultra busy. I offered to take him out to lunch for an interview, but he was too pressed for time. Not only did he have urgent obligations to attend to at the clinic, but also he couldn't work late because of a family obligation.

Dr. Douwes skipped his lunch and invited me into his office to interview him. He's a warm and friendly man, like a favorite grandfather.

In fact, Dr. Douwes is the "grandfather" of German cancer doctors: he taught many of the doctors I interviewed at other clinics, including Dr. Herzog, Dr. Migeod, and Dr. Wehner.

I asked Dr. Douwes if he could tell me three or four stories of patients who had come to him with "terminal" cancer who are now well.

Without batting an eye, he replied, "I have more than four. I could give you 400." He told me that many Americans come to his clinic for cancer treatment: "There are about 10 Americans here now. You can interview them."

Dr. Douwes proudly showed me his bestselling book *Hope for Prostate Disease: The New Treatment without a Knife*.

Regarding prostate cancer, he said, "There's no surgery and no biopsy. We can diagnose prostate cancer 100 percent without a biopsy. We can offer treatment without a knife. The patient gets to keep his prostate. We get rid of the cancer through hyperthermia in conjunction with low-dose chemotherapy."

Dr. Douwes further explained, "Our prostate cancer patients live as long as patients who have surgery but with a better quality of life: No incontinence or impotence! The treatment is tolerated well with little or no side effects. They enjoy a good quality of life. We have many such cases. You can interview some of them.

"When the patient comes, we do detox, detox, detox plus supplementation of vitamins and minerals. Then we destroy the cancer with low-dose chemo and hyperthermia. After tumor destruction we use chelation to get rid of toxic metals that are liberated from the tumor. This works beautifully. Then we send patients home with a six-week supply of metronomic chemo [a continuous supply of low dose chemo taken orally]. I don't know of any cancer that doesn't react to this kind of treatment."

Regarding brain cancer, Dr. Douwes said his clinic is very successful: "We at least triple the life expectancy. We lose some patients, but we've saved many."

Nine-year-old Jessika got rid of her brain cancer at St. George

Dr. Douwes wasn't just blowing smoke when he told me his clinic was good at getting rid of brain cancer. He told me the story of a nine-year-old girl from Stuttgart named Jessika who came to his clinic in 1999.

Jessika had a huge tumor on the right side of her brain that caused her to be paralyzed on the left side of her body. Today she's completely free of her cancer. Her mind is normal so she's able to finish school. Dr. Douwes said it's delightful to see Jessika developing into a lovely young woman. Sadly, she still has paralysis on the left side of her body because the cancer inflicted so much damage, but the cancer itself is long gone.

I interviewed two American patients from Oklahoma who were there because of word-of-mouth advertising from a satisfied patient who had gotten rid of his brain cancer at St. George over five years earlier.

Surprisingly, Dr. Douwes learned oncology in America in the 1970s. That means he learned all about the American cut-burn-poison method of treating cancer.

Dr. Douwes is reluctant to give chemo. He says, "I give it as much as necessary but as little as possible – along with complementary things such as nutrition, orthomolecular therapy (supplements), immune boosting therapy, and hormone balancing."

Why so many American men are growing breasts!

A big health problem today is that many men have no sex drive, and they're growing breasts ("man boobs")! Such men desperately need a hormonal tune-up, and many come to St. George just for the hormone balancing – not for anything having to do with cancer. Dr. Douwes is glad to oblige them with the necessary hormonal tune-up.

During my tour of St. George I saw the rooms where the various therapies take place, including:

- Detoxification procedures, including a foot bath detox
- Electro Dermal Screening (a non-invasive diagnostic technique using acupressure points)
- Infusion therapy (the IV room)
- Lymphatic massage
- Colonic hydrotherapy
- Magnetic field therapy
- Therapeutic mud treatment
- Relaxation techniques
- Therapeutic salt-water baths
- Far infrared sauna
- Hyperthermia (whole body and local)

I also saw a patient room, which was quite pleasant, and St. George's chapel. In St. George's spacious and comfortable lounge I interviewed three of the English-speaking patients.

The doctor told Debbie: "Get your will in order: you have 3 months"

The first American I interviewed was 37-year-old Debbie, a mother of three from Tulsa, Oklahoma. She told me that five years ago a mole on the back of her leg, which she'd had from birth, changed. She had it removed because it had turned into melanoma.

Sometime later, Debbie noticed a lump near the scar on her calf and another lump on her right shoulder. Both were melanoma, and she had them removed. Then she started getting new tumors on her chest and breast. She also had tumors on her adrenal gland and on the sacral nerve.

In America she was treated with radiation on the sacral tumor, which she said gave her some pain relief. She also took an oral chemotherapy drug.

Debbie learned about St. George from a cousin whose friend had actually gone there six years earlier for brain cancer. He'd never undergone any other treatments, and he remained cancer free. Once a month he was going in for an IV vitamin C infusion.

Let me just take a break from Debbie's story to point out something important: Anyone who reads this book and as a result goes to Germany to get rid of cancer should remember the last sentence in the previous paragraph: it bears repeating that the long-term brain cancer survivor continues receiving an IV vitamin C infusion from an American doctor each month.

You don't just go to Germany and get rid of your cancer in two or three weeks and come home "cured," never having to worry about cancer again. That's not the way it is.

After you get rid of your cancer, you have to commit yourself to an ongoing program of some kind, including permanent lifestyle changes, to keep the cancer from sneaking back. The monthly program of intravenous vitamin C is a smart strategy. The proof is in the pudding. Nothing succeeds like success, and you, too, can be a success story.

Now back to Debbie's story.

At the famous M.D. Anderson cancer hospital in Houston, doctors recommended that Debbie do an aggressive program of chemotherapy. She says, "I didn't want to do that. It wasn't for me." She did 10 radiation treatments, but when they were over she had to decide what she was going to do next.

When she told one doctor she didn't want to do his chemotherapy program, he washed his hands of her. Debbie says, "He told me to get my will in order and said I had one to three months to live. He wanted me to go home and die."

But Debbie told me, "I have three kids. I need to live!"

When we spoke, she had been at St. George for almost three weeks. When she first arrived, the clinic even sent a driver to pick her up at the airport. She figured she'd probably come back for a follow up visit "in a few months." Thus, there was no question in her mind that the doctor who predicted she had "one to three months to live" was just plain wrong.

St. George instructed Debbie to eliminate as much sugar as possible and to eat lots of fruits and vegetables. Honey is permitted.

She describes St. George as "wonderful. I'm so impressed. I had no idea what I was coming into. I did read one bad thing online. Someone had had a bad experience at this clinic. But you can have a bad experience anywhere."

Debbie said, "I know my body is very sick inside, but I really believe it's becoming well. The first week was mostly local hyperthermia to the adrenal and sacral area. I did that every day alternating for an hour except for the weekend. I also have magnetic field therapy. This increases oxygen in the cells and promotes healing. I love it because I get a little nap. I do that every day." A nurse leads relaxation exercises, which Debbie said she had done six times. "I love it. It helps me get focused and concentrate on what I have to do." She said she also does meditation exercises, and "that's what my day consists of."

The first time Debbie was treated with whole body hyperthermia it made her feel "crummy" for a few days. They had told her to expect that. But she told me that when she had it again the previous Monday, "I didn't feel bad."

Debbie said she'd had colonic hydrotherapy twice at St. George and was scheduled for another colonic the next day. She intends to keep up a program of regular colonics when she gets home as part of her ongoing lifestyle change.

I asked Debbie what she would say to Americans with cancer who might be thinking about going to St. George. She said, "This is one of the best facilities anybody could ever come to. The staff is wonderful. Dr. Douwes and the other physicians are wonderful. They're the best!"

Given just two years to live, Scott is living his bonus years

The next English-speaking patient I interviewed was Scott, an American professor of psychology who has been living in Europe for the last 18 years. His permanent home is in Spain. Scott was at St. George because of a relapse of his cancer.

Scott found out he had cancer exactly four years ago. He was diagnosed in London, and he told me that British doctors put together a conventional treatment plan for him that looked "horrible." They told him, "You've got to start chemo tomorrow!" They were pushing hard, trying to hustle him into their program. He refused.

He was diagnosed with a rare form of non-Hodgkins lymphoma. Conventional doctors consider it "incurable." The life expectancy of patients with this kind of cancer, according to conventional doctors, is two years. By that yardstick, Dr. Douwes has already helped Scott get two bonus years.

Scott told Dr. Douwes: "Look, I want 20 more years." The doctor replied, "We're working on it."

Word of mouth advertising from two satisfied patients influenced Scott to come to St. George for cancer treatment. He has been through a range of integrative treatments including whole body hyperthermia with low dose chemo. He said, "When I told my conventional folks how much chemo it was, they said, 'Wow! That's like nothing. Do it. It won't hurt you.'"

His first week of treatment focused on nutrition and boosting the immune system: magnetic field therapy, ozone therapy, oxygen therapy, and a daily infusion alternating between vitamin C and selenium. He got colonic hydrotherapy once a week, just before each session of whole body hyperthermia. And in Spain he continues his colonics, a wise practice.

Scott told me that Dr. Douwes has him on lots of nutritional supplements. And he said St. George has a "fabulous" psychologist who's skilled at counseling and gives the patients major support. He said she's a "lovely, talented person."

Regarding Dr. Douwes, Scott told me, "He's brilliant. I love how he pulls out your medical record, and you tell him four things, and he tells you the whole story of your life – past, present, and future – and it makes sense. It blows you away. He's on top of everything. The doctors are all talented, amazing, and bright. The nurses are outstanding."

Dale from Oklahoma can't say enough good things about St. George

We also interviewed Dale and Nancy from a suburb just outside Oklahoma City. They found out about St. George from their son, who lived next door to someone who had been a patient there.

Dale and Nancy said the patient was treated at St. George for brain cancer and had been in remission for five years. Debbie had told me a few minutes earlier about a similar case in which the man had been free from brain cancer for six years. Considering that they're all from Oklahoma, they could well be talking about the same patient.

April 4, 2004, was a day Dale will never forget. On that day he found out he had "the big C" – cancer. He had a particularly aggressive form of prostate cancer. Not too surprisingly, a surgeon recommended surgery. (When the only tool at hand is a hammer, everything tends to look like a nail.) As a result, he had his prostate cut out.

But Dale's cancer returned at the site of the scar tissue from his surgery.

Dale told me, "I took whole body hyperthermia last Monday [four days ago]. It was a tough day and a tough night, and it was tough for a couple of days after that. Today [Thursday] is the first day I felt pretty good, really. My body's coming back to normal. If that's all you have to do to live a normal life and to extend your life and have a good quality of life, it's worth it."

Regarding the food, Dale said, "The food is healthy. I like McDonald's, so I'll have to learn a different way of living. In a few days I'll get food recommendations to use at home. They don't allow sugar here. Instead, they use some kind of brown sugar but not the kind we have in America. It's more of a health food sugar. The cakes are made with applesauce for sweetener. And salt and pepper are hard to find here. They use sea salt. They stay away from the red meats."

Dale summed up his feeling about St. George, saying, "I couldn't say enough nice things about the four doctors. They're very well trained. Very helpful. Very caring. All their staff is, too."

American doctor recommended $100,000 chemo drug to Ron

On a subsequent visit to St. George I met Ron, a late-stage prostate cancer patient from Detroit. His American urologist recommended St. George because he had a prostate cancer patient who went there 12 years ago and was happy with his treatment. After Ron talked to that former cancer patient he decided that going to St. George was the right thing to do.

When Ron was being treated at the University of Michigan Hospital in Ann Arbor, doctors wanted to put him on high dose chemotherapy — a $100,000 treatment. Ron said no. His doctors tried to plug him into a clinical trial, but he told me, "I didn't want to be the guy who gets the placebo." Again, he said no. He wanted real treatment.

In fact, Ron never underwent any conventional treatment. And that gives him a better chance of beating his cancer because, high dose radiation and chemo can devastate the immune system.

At St. George, in addition to local hyperthermia to the prostate, Ron received two full-body hyperthermia treatments, and one more was scheduled when he and I spoke.

He told me, "Full body hyperthermia is a no-brainer because they put you under. All I remember is getting up in my room, and the next day I felt good. I've gained 8 pounds since I've been here. Food is completely different from what I normally eat, but I always find something I like."

Although Ron was fully insured for medical treatment in America, he decided to pay for the German treatment out of his own pocket, whether he gets any reimbursement or not. But Americans who go to Germany for cancer treatment have a good chance of getting their American health insurance to pay for a significant part of the medical costs, as I'll explain in a moment.

I asked Ron what he would tell Americans about St. George. "The clinic is first class," he replied. "I'm impressed with the people, the staff, the equipment. Getting to the clinic was quick and easy. They picked me up at the airport. The town's nice."

Near death, 29-year-old Chinese woman comes to St. George

In China, doctors gave no hope to a 29-year-old woman who was close to liver failure because of a massive tumor that had taken over four-fifths of her liver. She heard about St. George, and when she came to the clinic she was desperate, scared, and jaundiced.

Dr. Douwes told me that his Chinese patients are typically full of toxins from breathing bad air. He couldn't promise the lady results, but he put her through a rigorous detox program. Her jaundice got better, and the gigantic tumor shrank by a third after just three weeks. Her progress continued, and he sent her home with a normally functioning liver and very little tumor mass left.

Dr. Douwes said, "This case proves that people can get healthy again. It's a joy to see this."

How Dr. Douwes saved his son's life

Two of Dr. Douwes's children work at St. George: a daughter who's a dermatologist and a son who does CRS testing for cancer patients and Lyme disease patients.

The CRS device measures the patient's cells to see where the deficits are. Dr. Douwes's son showed me how the machine works. The patient's hand is placed on a laser device that measures metabolic substances found in the residue in skin cells. The device measures 300 different substances, and a computer calculates the results and generates a report. This report gives an overview of metabolic acidosis and regulation, immune defense, and regulation of immune function. It's a quick and thorough test.

The doctors at St. George use this tool to recommend an appropriate supplementation and eating plan. Then the test is repeated to see how well the recommendations are working. Dr. Douwes's son gave himself this test over a year before I interviewed him, and the results were appalling. He'd been constantly ill with colds and flu, he was acidic, and he looked worse than some of St. George's seriously ill cancer patients. Alarmed, he showed the results to his dad and said, "Look, we treat everybody. These test results are for me. Help me! I'm dying!"

Dr. Douwes gave his son advice about changing his eating plan, nutritional supplementation, and how to lose weight. He set his mind on improving his health and lost 80 pounds. He told me he'd recently repeated the CRS test, and the results were much better.

Regarding the best eating plan for cancer patients, Dr. Douwes said, "I'm not a fan of cancer diets. I'm only a fan of the right nutrition: no sugar, low carb, no red meat; poultry and fish are allowed, and also vegetables, vegetables, vegetables, either raw or cooked al dente [firm to the bite]. Vegetable juice, yes. Fruit, yes, but no fruit juice because of the sugar. Coconut oil is good for cooking. I don't like the ketogenic diet because of weight loss and because ketones can feed the tumor."

St. George offers a wide variety of lifesaving therapies

St. George claims to have the largest hyperthermia center in the world. It has four full-body hyperthermia machines and four local hyperthermia machines. In addition, it has three transurethral hyperthermia machines — a new therapy for prostate cancer.

St. George also has a remarkable record of treating breast cancer. One of the most effective therapies is Galvano therapy — a therapy developed by an Austrian physician but now used most extensively in China. Galvano therapy uses a carefully monitored dose of direct current to kill the cancer cells without causing discomfort.

St. George is one of two clinics I visited that uses a therapy developed to keep Soviet cosmonauts healthy: laser therapy by IV. I don't know how it works, but according to patients, it improves energy and makes them feel good.

Photodynamic therapy is another new treatment St. George offers. In this therapy the patient receives chlorophyll by IV, which locates the tumor. Then the tumor is exposed to laser light that destroys the cancer. Dr. Douwes said, "It's a mild treatment for those who are very sick. It's an easy-to-do method."

Detoxification: "You have to get the garbage out of your system"

Detoxification is job one, according to Dr. Douwes. He says the typical American cancer patient is constipated and full of toxicity from heavy metals, toxic organic substances, and prescription drugs.

"You have to get the garbage out of your system," said Dr. Douwes. Detoxification at St. George includes colonic hydrotherapy, coffee enemas, vitamin C by IV, lymphatic massage, far infrared saunas, chelation, and other therapies.

I met three other doctors at St. George: Dr. Georg Kroiss, Dr. Marian Reichel, and Dr. Gabriele Zabel. All of these doctors impressed me.

Dr. Kroiss spent 10 years at a clinic in Tanzania before coming to St. George, where he has been for several years. Until World War I, Tanzania was a German colony called German East Africa.

Dr. Reichel told me why St. George doesn't recommend cutting out the prostate, as American doctors routinely recommend. Not only can prostate removal cause impotence and incontinence, but there are other complications.

Ancient Chinese medicine regards the prostate as the "fire of life," explained Dr. Reichel. The prostate is the seat of male energy. Dr. Reichel said that when the prostate is removed, aging accelerates. A man's head may sink into his shoulders and he may start to shuffle with a little stoop. Dr. Reichel said he can tell at a glance when a man has had his prostate taken out. I found that remarkable – and a powerful argument for keeping your prostate unless its removal is absolutely necessary.

100 percent success rate with new prostate cancer treatment!

Dr. Douwes has demonstrated a 100 percent success rate with a revolutionary therapy for prostate cancer that saves the prostate.

He did a study on 123 prostate cancer patients. Over a one-week period the patients got two painless treatments of transurethral hyperthermia in addition to other out-patient therapies. Of the original 123 patients, 85 percent had no more cancer after 10 years. They didn't even have to see a urologist. The other 15 percent needed re-treatment, which was successful. Not one of these 123 patients died of cancer or had any complications related to the therapy. And they kept their prostates.

For example, an American pilot named Jeff Albulet underwent St. George's one-week program for his prostate cancer, which includes two transurethral hyperthermia treatments. Here's how he described it:

"The treatment was a breeze. I felt no pain at all. I had a treatment in the morning and played golf in the afternoon. Everyone at the hospital was so caring. The only side effects I have are positive. I no longer have to get up at night, and all my parts are functioning perfectly."

Dr. Douwes strongly believes that there's no need to remove, destroy, or compromise the prostate. Unlike conventional cancer treatments, prostate cancer treatment at St. George doesn't cause impotence or incontinence. He declares, "Local hyperthermia for prostate cancer is the answer!"

Because of his remarkable and pioneering accomplishments in integrative cancer treatment, Dr. Douwes was honored to be the first German to receive the Lifetime Achievement Award from the Academy of Comprehensive Integrative Medicine.

Dr. Douwes accidentally discovers a cure for Lyme disease

Lyme disease isn't just a problem in America. It's also a problem in Germany. Dr. Douwes accidentally discovered a cure for Lyme disease when he was treating two breast cancer patients in the year 2000. One lady was from Massachusetts, and the other was from Canada. In addition to breast cancer, they also had Lyme disease. Dr. Douwes was astonished when they came out of whole-body hyperthermia and remarked, independent of each other, "My Lyme symptoms are gone!"

Dr. Douwes figured he might be onto something, so he told his staff, "We should go after this!"

Dr. Douwes attended a medical conference in America about Lyme disease. An American doctor sitting next to him asked, "Why are you here?" Dr. Douwes replied, "I'm here to learn something about Lyme disease. I don't know much about it. I'm an oncologist."

The other doctor said, "I'm a cardiologist. I'm here because my wife, daughter, and son got infected during a vacation. My wife has been bedridden for two years. My daughter is a medical student but can't attend medical school anymore because she can't follow the lessons. My son, a violinist, can't play the violin anymore because he can't control his fingers.

"I'm going from conference to conference to find out if any treatment is available, but all I hear is 'antibiotics, antibiotics, antibiotics.' My wife and daughter have been on antibiotics for almost two years. Nothing helped my son. I'm desperate. I'm still going to these conferences hoping that someday I'll find something."

When Dr. Douwes told him about whole-body hyperthermia for Lyme disease at St. George, the cardiologist immediately said, "I'll send you my family!" Dr. Douwes replied, "I can't advise you to send your family because I can't promise that they'll be cured. I only have experience with giving hyperthermia to a few Lyme patients." The cardiologist said, "What can we lose?" So he brought his family to St. George.

At St. George the cardiologist's bedridden wife was cured and was able to return to work. His daughter was cured, finished medical school, and is now a practicing physician. His son was cured and is now a professor of music and the conductor of the college orchestra. Dr. Douwes told me, "That was 10 years years ago. It was a breakthrough for us."

Dr. Douwes improved his protocol for Lyme patients after he came across an article in a medical journal about how fever temperatures increase the effectiveness of antibiotics. The article said that increasing the fever by one degree Celsius increases the antibiotic activity 16-fold. The article recommended temperatures that matched what Dr. Douwes was already using in his whole-body hyperthermia treatments.

During whole-body hyperthermia for Lyme patients, Dr. Douwes started adding antibiotics at 40 degrees Celsius (104 degrees Fahrenheit) and increased the temperature to a plateau of 41.6 degrees (106.9 degrees Fahrenheit). He told me, "I'm so happy with this treatment," which he calls Antibiotic Augmented Thermal Regulation.

Another breakthrough happened when an Australian Lyme patient came to St. George and returned home cured. A news story about this man's recovery appeared on Australian television, and that's when St. George's Lyme disease treatment program skyrocketed. St. George now gets about five inquiries a day from Australia about Lyme disease, primarily from the Melbourne and Perth areas.

Vineyard owner says, "Help me, or I'll shoot myself!"

One Lyme patient told Dr. Douwes, "You can't imagine the pain. My life is over. I can't go to my vineyards anymore. If you don't help me, I'm going to shoot myself." After the first hyperthermia treatment at St. George he was completely pain free. When he returned home, he called Dr. Douwes and said, "You gave me my life back." For a Christmas present he sent two cases of his finest wine to St. George.

These days, about half of St. George's patients – 700 to 800 a year – are there for Lyme disease. Ironically, Dr. Douwes's Lyme disease protocol may eventually overshadow his remarkable influence as a pioneer in integrative cancer care!

About two-thirds of St. George's Lyme patients are able to go back to a normal life. Of the other third, most have a fair result but still suffer because of being confined to a wheelchair for so long. For about 10 to 15 percent of Lyme patients, the treatment made little difference, despite Dr. Douwes's best efforts. He told me, "In medicine there are no guarantees. I do the best I can, and I'm helping a lot of people. It's not possible to please everyone."

Each year St. George gets money from the government of Bavaria to improve the hospital. The government supports it because St. George has become famous and has attracted a large number of medical tourists.

Cost of treatment at St. George

Cancer treatment at St. George requires a deposit of 21,000 Euros in advance. But another deposit might be required at the end of the second week of treatment. There are extra charges for some of the therapies. Each case is different, and before you go to St. George, you should request an estimate of costs based on the treatment plan the doctor proposes.

For early-stage prostate carcinoma, St. George offers a one-week package for just 6,000 Euros. This includes remarkably effective treatments of local hyperthermia to the prostate at 50 degrees Celsius. These treatments kill the cancer, awaken the immune system, improve urination, and leave the prostate unharmed!

The clinic also offers a one-week 4,000 Euro package to treat BPH (enlarged prostate) using local hyperthermia. The clinic has found that this treatment gives the best chance of complete recovery.

Lyme disease treatment costs are different. The first two weeks of treatment, which includes hyperthermia, antibiotics, and detox, costs 15,000 Euros. Repairing damaged systems requires more time and expense. (For example, Lyme disease causes thyroid problems, adrenal problems, and sexual problems such as no menstruation for young women whose hormone levels drop to the level of post-menopausal women.) Each case is different.

St. George works with a billing company called American Medical Health Alliance in Houston, Texas, to persuade American health insurance companies to cover the treatments in Germany.

St. George says that American Medical Health Alliance has "a success rate of getting claims paid by your insurance company of 85 to 90 percent." In other words 85 to 90 percent of insured Americans get some reimbursement from their insurance company while 10 to 15 percent of patients get no reimbursement.

Patients normally come with a friend or relative, and the clinic charges a nominal fee for room and board for the relative. Outpatients can stay at the nearby Lindners Hotel, which offers a special rate for St. George patients. Other housing options are available. If a patient room at St. George isn't needed for an inpatient, an outpatient may occupy it.

A friendly and compassionate staff member named Frederika Montpetit is the first contact person for international patients. She tells the patients what kind of records St. George needs to see, and she coordinates everything with the doctor. She's with the patient through the entire process from the time they arrive until they go back home.

Patients don't have the feeling that they're sick and in a clinic because St. George doesn't look or seem like a hospital. It looks more like a hotel.

o get to St. George

. George is simple. All you have
unich, and the clinic will send
you up. That's it! Some patients
like to travel on the weekend. For example, it
only takes an hour by train to get to Munich.
Patients can also sign up for day trips by bus.

Contact information:

Klinik St. Georg (St. George Hospital)

Rosenheimer Straße 6-8 83043
Bad Aibling, Germany

Head physician: Dr. Friedrich R. Douwes

Website: www.klinik-st-georg.de

e-mail: info@klinik-st-georg.de

Phone: 011-49-08061-398-0

Fax: 011-49-08061-398-454

Chapter Twelve

Dr. Axel Weber's Klinik Marinus am Stein in Brannenburg

A surgeon who recommends *against* cancer surgery?

At the very top of the website of Dr. Axel Weber, M.D., is this historic motto of the entire medical profession: *Primum non nocere*! The English translation for this Latin motto is: First do no harm!

That motto is the guiding principle of Dr. Weber's Klinik Marinus am Stein, which means Marinus in Stone. This motto explains why, even though he's trained as a surgeon, he usually recommends *against* surgery. If surgery would harm the cancer patient, Dr. Weber (pronounced "Vay-ber," which means "Weaver" in German) believes no doctor should do it, period.

Why should a patient have surgery if there's a better way to get rid of cancer?

Dr. Weber's clinic is located amidst the picturesque Bavarian Alps. And you wouldn't believe what a charming village Brannenburg is. To preserve the charm of the village, the municipal building codes are strict.

In 1999, when Dr. Weber bought the "building" that became his clinic, it was a dilapidated shell consisting of four walls. There weren't even any floors. He preserved the original four walls but otherwise rebuilt it from the ground up.

Within just six months the intimate 26-bed clinic was open for business! The clinic has 18 rooms in the main house and eight more in the guesthouse. It looks charming from the outside and beautiful on the inside. Besides patients

in residence, the clinic normally has 10 to 15 outpatients who stay at a nearby hotel or bed & breakfast.

Dr. Weber's wife gave me a tour. She is also a physician (an anesthesiologist). And the clinic's third physician is a general practitioner.

Here are some of the therapies the clinic offers:

- Whole-body hyperthermia with low-dose chemo
- Local hyperthermia
- Magnetic-field therapy
- Detoxification procedures including the foot bath detox
- Oxygen therapy
- Ozone therapy
- Mistletoe therapy
- Intravenous vitamin C and selenium
- Foot reflexology
- Electro-dermal screening (a non-invasive diagnostic technique using acupressure points)
- Acupuncture
- Colonic hydrotherapy

The clinic includes a room where Dr. Weber occasionally performs small surgeries when necessary. He performs no major surgeries or abdominal surgeries.

I personally saw Dr. Axel Weber assisting a patient up some stairs. When would you ever see that in an American hospital?

When I sat down with Dr. Weber for an interview, he told me, "We're a little clinic specializing in cancer treatment. In cancer, the whole body is ill. You can't just cut off a breast and pretend everything's O.K. You must treat the whole patient. That's why we use a combination therapy for the whole body."

Why surgery so often fails to get rid of cancer

As for surgery, he stated, "It's better for the patient to avoid surgery if at all possible. As a surgeon, I usually recommend *against* surgery. Unless you get at the *cause* of the cancer, you'll get metastasis. It's not enough just to get rid of the tumor. You have to get rid of the metastasized cells, and that requires treating the whole body."

Like the other German cancer clinics I visited, Dr. Weber uses a combination of natural medicine and conventional medicine. If the natural treatment isn't enough to do the job, he suggests low-dose chemo.

Without a doubt, Dr. Weber is an expert in hyperthermia, an important part of the whole treatment plan. He founded the Hyperthermia Society of Germany, and he's given 14,000 hyperthermia treatments since then.

Dr. Weber told me, "At our little clinic we have an outstanding relationship with the patients. And this is important." He said there's little or no staff turnover at the clinic. This stability fosters a close relationship with the patients.

When I asked him to tell me about patients who'd come to him with "terminal" cancer and who had a successful outcome, he reached for his thick scrapbook.

61-year-old lady avoids disfiguring facial surgery

Back in 1995 – five years before he opened his new clinic – a 61-year-old lady came to Dr. Weber with skin cancer (melanoma). Her doctor had recommended drastic surgery that would've horribly disfigured her eye and ear. She was desperate. Her cancer was ugly. It looked bad and even smelled bad.

Dr. Weber recommended against surgery and instead treated her successfully with his other methods. He said, "She still lives today."

Turning to another page in his scrapbook, Dr. Weber showed me a shocking photo of an ugly case of breast cancer. In a heartbeat, conventional doctors would have recommended a mastectomy (cutting off the breast), but not Dr. Weber. Without chemo or surgery, he helped this woman (born in 1952) overcome her cancer. As proof, he showed us a photo of her improvement.

Dr. Weber showed us similar photos of breast cancer in a woman born in 1951. Her tumor was large, and it had metastasized. With neither surgery nor radiation, he helped this woman, too, get rid of her cancer. The "before" and "after" photos proved the effectiveness of his methods.

Surgery for prostate cancer? Dr. Weber insists, "Never, never, never, NEVER!"

At Klinik Marinus, Dr. Weber treats many patients with prostate cancer, but never with surgery: "Never, never, never, NEVER!" When a man's prostate is surgically removed, he explained, "30 out of 100 will die within 10 years."

It's too bad actor Robert De Niro didn't go to Dr. Weber's clinic instead of paying an American hospital $250,000 to have his prostate cut out.

A man born in 1937 came to the clinic when it first opened in 2000. He had severe prostate cancer. His PSA score was off the charts at 5,310. The following week, it was down to 4,300. The week after that it was down to 3,500 – a 2,000-point drop in three weeks. The cancer had metastasized to his bones. Now, though his PSA is still higher than normal, it's down to 25.

Dr. Weber says the PSA score is "only a number on a piece of paper."

The clinic also has great success with bladder cancer, liver cancer, blood cancer, Hodgkin's, and colon carcinoma.

The clinic doesn't accept children as patients. If you're looking for a clinic that accepts children, see the chapters about the Hufeland Klinik and Dr. Herzog's Fachklinik.

Dr. Weber told me he wants to help many more patients, but he doesn't want a bigger clinic. He believes he can best serve his patients by limiting the number to about 25 at any one time. And he's eager to accept more English-speaking cancer patients.

A picture is worth a thousand words

Lastly, Dr. Weber gave me a reprint of an article about his clinic from the August/September, 2003, issue of a German health magazine called *Bio*. I can't read German, but a picture is worth 1,000 words.

On page 42, a series of three photos shows a lady with a grotesque, ugly tumor on her ear lobe and upper jaw. The angry red tumor – bigger than a golf ball – looks like a deformed, mutant vegetable. The second photo shows the tumor virtually gone, though the tissues look bruised. The third photo shows normal skin coloration. Remarkable! In the USA, this woman probably would have undergone drastic, disfiguring surgery – plus radiation and chemo.

On page 44, a series of four photos shows a woman with a massive, unsightly cancer on her left breast. Each subsequent photo shows improvement, and the last one shows normal skin coloration. A similar series of photos of another former breast cancer patient appears on page 45.

When I returned to the clinic for another visit, Dr. Weber told me that quite a few patients had come there as a result of *German Cancer Breakthrough*. He said, "One of them is here from Oklahoma and would be glad to speak to you." I'll describe my interview with him in a moment.

Dr. Weber said that new patients had come not just from America but also from Australia, Canada, South Africa, Greece, and Romania.

Dr. Weber uses the recently developed procedure called transurethral local hyperthermia, administered through a catheter, to treat prostate cancer. This is a simple, effective, inexpensive way to get rid of prostate cancer. It only takes one week, and there are no side effects.

Here's how it works. Dr. Weber inserts a catheter slowly and carefully into the urethra. Because of a local anesthetic, there is no pain. Once inserted, a radio wave from an electrode heats up the prostate from the inside out. The electrode is actually *in* the prostate, right where the cancer is. The electrode reaches a heat of 50 degrees Celsius (122 degrees Fahrenheit) and maintains that heat for two hours. Then the catheter is removed. The patient gets two of these treatments within one week, and then he can go home cancer free.

One eating plan doesn't fit all

Dr. Weber commented on the German tradition of offering a little cake to the patients in the afternoon – a tradition that several of Germany's top cancer clinics observe. Referring to his clinic, he said, "We have a home atmosphere. It's a nice house. I want the patients to be happy. The body wants a little cake with sugar. It's not healthy, but it's good for the patient's spirit.

"In the last 25 years I haven't seen a diet that was so good that it applies to all patients. Gerson is hard to do. Some diets say 'no dairy' but Budwig requires cottage cheese. The Coy diet recommends steak every day and eating lots of beef with few vegetables. Others say 'no beef.' I don't know. Nobody knows. Love your body and ask your body, 'What do you want,' and then give it some – not too much but in moderation. A beer or a little wine can lift a patient's spirit. It's good for the soul and good for health, but don't drink three liters! Some people say, 'no glucose!' But you need glucose for your brain and for your muscles.

"I don't say you must not eat sugar, and I don't say you must not drink alcohol. Just not too much. Be moderate."

He recommends the Budwig anti-cancer mixture in the morning: flax oil mixed with quark. (Americans who use the Budwig diet use cottage cheese with the flax oil as a substitute for quark.) The Budwig protocol is an excellent recommendation not only to help get rid of cancer but to keep it away. For those who want to eat the Budwig mixture at home, see chapter two about Lothar Hirneise's 3E center near Stuttgart.

Another powerful remedy that Dr. Weber uses is laetrile, the powerful anti-cancer substance that Mexico's top cancer clinics use. But he says, "I have no miracle. The patient must believe in the treatment plan, as I do, and then we can move forward together. Every patient has a chance when they believe inside that they'll have success."

Dr. Weber urges patients to love their body and to speak to their cancer. He tells cancer patients: "The cancer is part of your body. Speak with your cancer every day when you go to bed. Put your hand on the cancer and say, 'Hey, Cancer. We've been together for a long time. But now it's time for you to leave my body. If you kill me, you'll die, too.' Why not? It's very important. I have time for the patient. I have no psychologists here. They come to me every day. When they have a problem, they can talk to me about it. The patients must feel that I'm here for *them*."

After visiting with Dr. Weber, I met the prostate cancer patient from Oklahoma, Mike, who was there with his wife. Here's what Mike said:

"I'm fairly healthy. I don't catch colds. But I got prostate cancer a year and a half ago. My urologist immediately suggested surgery. But the cancer was slow-growing, so surgery didn't make sense to me. I didn't want treatments with complications and side effects, so I opted against doing any conventional treatment.

"I saw an advertisement for *German Cancer Breakthrough*. I ordered it. I read it. I loved what I read. I decided to come to Germany to get what I consider the pre-eminent treatment in the world, which is here. It's our first trip to Germany. I can tell you I love it. I take a walk outside, and it's bucolic. I mean, there are cows up there with the bells on them. The green fields. The Alps. It's truly, truly marvelous. And this is a very healing place. I'm leaving tomorrow. Dr. Weber said I only needed a week of treatment. This is a great clinic, and Dr. Weber is a great doctor."

"My doctors are *here*"

I asked Mike what his doctor back home is going to say about his treatment in Germany. He replied, "I have my doctors *here*. I'm done with those doctors in America."

I asked Mike, "Could you please describe the trans-urethral hyperthermia treatment of the prostate? Was it comfortable? Uncomfortable?"

Here's how Mike described it: "I've been through it twice this week. It's a two-hour treatment. The only discomfort, and it's minor, is the insertion of the catheter. That's the same approximate discomfort that anyone would have with any catheter. You just lay there, and the doctor puts the catheter in. He adjusts the machine, and heats it up, and then raises the temperature. And they constantly check on you to make sure you're okay and give you some water to drink.

"What I did yesterday is I just meditated during the two hours. For healing, for relaxation. And the time goes by quickly when you do something like that. Not a problem. Dr. Weber explains everything to you. I never had a catheter before, so I didn't know what to expect. But he's so good that you're not apprehensive. And it goes very, very well. After my treatment I actually *feel* different around the prostate. Now it feels like the cancer's gone."

Mike's wife commented, "One thing that surprised Mike is how much they touch him, I mean, physically touch him. Doctors come down here throughout the day just to see how he's feeling, to see if he's having any problems. This caring is just not seen in the states. We just don't have doctors like this.

"In America, they never ask how you're feeling. And that's what we've noticed from the very beginning is just the warmth, the care, they touch you physically. The nurse walks by and puts her hand on Mike's shoulder. They're not getting all 'gloved up' as if they're scared to touch you. They're not doing that. It's just different."

I asked Mike what he would say to an American cancer patient thinking about going to a German clinic. He replied, "Even though there may be some apprehension, come! Because it's too good. The treatment's too good here. And once you're here, apprehension goes away. You just have to take the plunge and make the leap of faith, and it works."

Mike asked me to autograph his copy of *German Cancer Breakthrough*. I was glad to do so, after which he shook my hand and said, "Thank you for saving my life."

While touring the clinic I met Mario S. from Canada who was having transurethral hyperthermia. Mario told me, "I've read your book. I'm pleased to meet you. It's a great thing you're doing. It's fantastic." I replied, "I think you're in the right place." He said, "I am. Absolutely!"

I also met an American from Panama whose wife was being treated for cancer. They had read my book. He told me, "You probably couldn't say enough good about this clinic. I think the key to the whole thing is that people have to be open-minded enough to understand the benefits of the whole health care system here. People are brought up as youngsters to trust the doctor. You must obey whatever the doctor says. To break that mold and go to a clinic in Germany is difficult for most people. They believe in the American medical profession."

The most amazing story I heard at the clinic was from Jeffrey, an American living in Switzerland. Conventional doctors in Switzerland had given him a terrible prognosis, telling him, "You have Stage Four cancer of the liver and pancreas."

They wanted to do a biopsy, but Jeffrey's gut told him to take a pass. A nurse called his home and asked why he cancelled the appointment for the biopsy. His wife told her, "He wants to do alternative care." The nurse replied, "I understand, and I agree."

Patient thanks me for writing *German Cancer Breakthrough*

He did some research, and he found my book *German Cancer Breakthrough*. He told me, "It's the best money I've ever spent on a book! After reading it I ultimately chose this clinic, and I'm very happy to be here. This is the third time I've come, and it's not because I'm getting worse but because I'm getting better. When I returned home after the first round of treatment, I was virtually a new person, and I became better and better.

"And then I went back to the Swiss hospital for a CT scan, which showed that the tumors had shrunk by about a third. My cancer markers had also declined significantly, and my blood results were getting better. I came back to the clinic for two more weeks to continue the process. Three months later I came back for another two weeks. The tumors keep shrinking and dying.

"It was divine intervention that I avoided a biopsy and conventional treatment. I have a good quality of life. I don't miss out on anything. In Switzerland they told me, 'You have three months to live.' If I'd taken chemo and radiation, I probably would've died after three months."

Jeffrey reiterated that *German Cancer Breakthrough* is "the best book I've ever bought."

More patient feedback about Dr. Weber's clinic

I sent out an e-mail to everyone who bought the first edition of *German Cancer Breakthrough*, requesting feedback – positive or negative – from customers who actually went to one of the clinics I recommended. Five customers gave me feedback about Dr. Weber's clinic. They were all positive.

One of these satisfied customers, Dr. Rainer Grundl from Melbourne, Australia, avoided major abdominal surgery for his stage four, advanced colorectal cancer by going to Dr. Weber's clinic. Dr. Grundl is a practicing homeopath. He wrote, "My wife and I stayed at Dr. Weber's clinic for 15 days. The best decision I ever made. I had local hyperthermia, a number of biological treatments such as ozone therapy by infusions every second day, hyperthermia every day for one hour, magnetic field therapy, infusions including selenium, vitamin C on alternative days and a number of immune stimulating therapies. In addition, I had localized cryosurgery (using a form of ice) therapies whereby the cancer was directly treated under anaesthesia.

"Dr. Weber and his staff, including his wife, who is also the anaesthetist, the nurses and administrative staff were just marvelous individuals. It is their professionalism, together with their considerate attitude, treating patients as individuals – all of this creates an atmosphere conducive to treatment as well as recovery. It was a delight to be there, almost feeling somewhat sad having to leave there." When Dr. Grundl returned home, tests indicated that no

cancer cells were detectable.

Three different customers also gave the clinic glowing recommendations:

"I cannot say enough good things about this man and his wife along with their staff."

"The care was second to none. Dr. Weber and his wife are two of the most caring people that I've ever had the pleasure to meet."

"I was very impressed with Dr. Weber's clinic."

Cost of treatment at Klinik Marinus am Stein

Patients at Klinik Marinus am Stein pay 370 Euros per day for a single room, 320 Euros per day for a double room. This price includes everything except medication for cancer patients. Drugs cost extra. With all of the therapies including hyperthermia, the costs are about 5,000 to 5,500 Euros per week.

Patients usually come with a companion who shares the patient's room. The charge for the companion is 80 Euros per day, which includes room and board.

The cost for outpatients is approximately 3,000 to 3,500 Euros per week.

How to get to Klinik Marinus am Stein

To get to Klinik Marinus am Stein, simply fly into Munich airport, and someone from the clinic will pick you up and give you door-to-door service free of charge.

If you're looking for an intimate clinic that gives lots of personal attention, this clinic certainly qualifies.

If you like skiing, you're only 20 minutes from the lifts. Granted, most cancer patients aren't going to want to ski, but the loved one or friend who accompanies the patient may want to hit the slopes. And even if you don't ski, it's pleasant to be in the Bavarian Alps.

You're just a five-minute drive from a Therme (spa) at the town of Bad Feilnbach. And the wonderful new Therme at Bad Aibling isn't much farther down the road.

The clinic offers the use of some bicycles; indeed, cycling in the open air is wonderful exercise – and fun. If it's been a long time since you've ridden a bike, it'll make you feel like a kid again!

If you're there in the summer, you can also swim in the nearby lakes. The water temperature reaches a pleasant 25 degrees Celsius, which is 77 degrees Fahrenheit. The village is charming, and the clinic is right next to a mountain.

Contact information:

Klinik Marinus am Stein

Biberstraße 30
83098 Brannenburg, Germany

Contact: Dr. Axel Weber

Website: www.klinik-marinus.de (The clinic is in the process of creating an English website, which might or might not be online by the time you read this.)

e-mail: info@klinik-marinus.de

Phone: 011-49-8034-908-0

Fax: 011-49-8034-908-299

Chapter Thirteen

Dr. Wilfried Stücker's IOZK Clinic in Cologne

The Immunologic Oncology Center in Cologne (Immunologisch Onkologisches Zentrum, Köln) is abbreviated IOZK.

Although IOZK's founder Dr. Wilfried Stücker is a naturopathic doctor, he doesn't describe his clinic as "holistic" or "alternative." Rather, he says it's solidly based on science. He focuses like a laser beam on the patient's immune system and how to boost it so that it can mop up cells that are abnormal or malignant. I interviewed Dr. Stücker and his colleague Dr. Tobias Sprenger, M.D.

Dr. Stücker has a good grasp of English, but Dr. Sprenger did most of the talking because he speaks English with complete fluency.

In Dr. Stücker's view, cancer is essentially an immune deficiency disease. To prevent, control, or cure cancer, the immune system is crucial. What the immune system needs in order to find and kill cancer cells is enough information about the target cells that need to be killed. If an abnormal cell sneaks past the immune system and starts multiplying, cancer can become a problem.

A strong immune system differentiates between the body's own cells and alien invaders – and also between harmless cells and dangerous cells. Cancer cells aren't invaders from outside the body but rather are produced by the patient's own body, but they're dangerous. These abnormal cells sometimes use a "tumor escape mechanism" to hide from the immune system.

Dr. Stücker wants the patient's own immune system to identify, attack, and kill the abnormal cells – a strategy that interests few conventional cancer doctors. Conventional therapies that cut, burn, or poison the cancer out of the patient's body do nothing to change the conditions that caused the body to produce the cancer in the first place. Chemotherapy and radiation indiscriminately attack both healthy and abnormal cells.

Furthermore, conventional therapy ignores an important fact: cancer stem cells have all the information necessary to grow a new tumor, and they can easily carry this information to other parts of the body and sprout new cancer cells. That's why cancer so often returns after conventional therapy. Sometimes cancer returns right after the therapy. In other cases, it may come back years later.

Dr. Sprenger remarked, "The concepts of traditional oncology are comparatively stupid. We're trying to beat these doctors with their own weapons by being better than they are and by applying new scientific evidence faster and better than they do. If the immune system is strengthened and educated to recognize the cancer cells as an enemy that needs to be destroyed, the immune system by itself can kill the bad cells."

IOZK's goal is to educate the patient's immune system so that it retains a memory and will be able to recognize cancer cells indefinitely in the future. Dr. Sprenger said, "Some conventional oncologists don't like this idea because it's the best tool you can get! We make our own vaccines here. It's an individualized treatment that requires a lot of man hours. The big drug companies don't like it because they don't make a profit on it. We teach the immune system to attack the body's own cancer cells."

When a cancer patient's immune system is properly educated, the tumor cells can no longer hide from the immune system but rather "wave a flag" and say, "I'm not doing well. Please kill me." The immune system promptly obliges. To beat cancer, it's not necessary to kill every single cancer cell in the patient's body. It's only necessary for the immune system to become strong enough to neutralize the tumors, turning them dormant.

Doctors Stücker and Sprenger help patients overcome death sentences

The doctors at IOZK have witnessed remarkable results with their immunotherapy, but the clinic has never done a double-blind placebo-controlled study to prove that immunotherapy gets better results than conventional therapy. That's because a placebo-controlled study of terminally ill patients would require the clinic to withhold immunotherapy from half of the patients, making it virtually certain that they would die within months. Would it be ethical to do a double-blind placebo-controlled study to test a therapy that's *known* to work? This would seem to be a cruel medical experiment. If I had terminal cancer and volunteered for a study on the effectiveness of immunotherapy, I would hate to find out I was in the placebo group.

Perhaps the strongest proof the clinic has for the effectiveness of its treatments is with glioblastoma brain cancer patients. This is the deadliest kind of brain cancer. Practically all glioblastoma patients who go through conventional therapy are dead within a year to 15 months. But the IOZK clinic has glio patients who are still alive after two, three, or five years. This survival can only be attributed to their unique combination of immunotherapies. It has nothing to do with luck, "spontaneous remission," or incorrect diagnosis.

Dr. Sprenger said, "We can't promise success, but we see many successful cases. In at least eight out of 10 patients we treat, we see the cancer-specific immune function get better. We see patients stay healthy. Some patients don't even tell their oncologist they're coming here. Some patients who come to us with a poor prognosis survive for five, eight, or 10 years or more."

Dr. Sprenger said the attitude of the medical community is starting to change toward the IOZK clinic. Ten years ago, conventional doctors warned cancer patients, "Don't do that! It's hocus pocus. They're just after your money." But when IOZK's patients have returned to their cancer doctors at universities in Salzburg, Paris, and elsewhere, these doctors ask: "Where did you go?" They can't argue with the results.

For example, a 75-year-old man underwent conventional therapy at his local university hospital for advanced, aggressive prostate cancer with metastasis to the bone. He had one foot in the grave, and his oncologist finally gave him the bad news: "We can't help you any more. We could do another round of chemo, but I don't recommend it." The pain in the patient's back was horrendous. He was desperate for pain relief and for a cure.

When he came to IOZK as a last resort, his PSA score was an astounding 233.8, even though he had already had a prostatectomy at the university hospital. But less than two months after starting immunotherapy at IOZK, his PSA dropped to less than one (0.8). After three months he was in complete remission. Dr. Sprenger said, "This case is a miracle. The guy sees us every six months to check his PSA level, which remains low."

Although immunotherapy saved this man's life, it couldn't undo the damage of the prostatectomy, which not only proved to be in vain but also led to permanent incontinence. The man is grateful to be alive but wishes he had started his cancer treatment at IOZK instead of doing conventional therapy first.

This case was published in the medical journal *Oncology Letters* 8: 2403-2406, 2014. You can find it on the journal's website in the December 2014 issue.

It's worth mentioning that IOZK also offers transurethral hyperthermia for prostate patients. This is an inexpensive method of applying local hyperthermia to the prostate. In cases where cancer is confined to the prostate, this is a safe and remarkably effective alternative to harsh or radical conventional methods of treatment. This therapy is also effective for benign prostate hyperplasia (BPH), which is also known as "enlarged prostate."

A 70-year-old housewife came to the IOZK clinic with severe breast cancer with metastasis to the liver. Conventional oncologists consider this incurable. The median survival time for breast cancer with metastasis to the liver is just six months without treatment. Survival time is 14 to 22 months with chemotherapy, but she declined chemotherapy because of the severe side effects that produce a miserable quality of life.

Instead, she chose immunotherapy at IOZK. Her treatments included the Newcastle disease virus, dendritic cell vaccinations, and hyperthermia. Her quality of life is excellent because these treatments have no severe side effects. Dr. Sprenger said, "This patient has never been hospitalized after the initial operation, which is unusual in cancer patients with metastases. She still sees us after five years and has immunotherapy every now and then."

This case was published in the medical journal *Immunotherapy* (2015) 7(8), 855-860. You can find this article on the *Immunotherapy* journal's website.

The Newcastle virus infiltrates cancer cells so they can be killed

Dr. Sprenger said, "We have an oncolytic virus that has the capacity to enter human tumor cells and kill them. One oncolytic virus – the Newcastle disease virus – is extraordinary. This virus is harmful to poultry but totally harmless for humans. The virus infiltrates cancer cells so they flash a danger signal at the immune system.

The Newcastle virus only infects the tumor cells, not normal cells. When cancer cells wave a red flag and beg the immune system to kill them, the immune system is easily able to distinguish between the healthy cells, which are left alone, and the abnormal cells, which are promptly killed.

If it's necessary to further boost the immune system, the clinic may also give patients moderate whole body hyperthermia with a plateau temperature between 38.5 and 40.5 degrees Celsius (101 to 105 degrees Fahrenheit). Local hyperthermia is applied directly to the tumor area. In addition to strengthening the immune system, hyperthermia kills or weakens cancer cells without harming normal cells.

Another strategy to kill tumor cells involves antigens. An antigen is a characteristic of a cell. The immune system needs to "see" a tumor-associated or tumor-specific antigen to know that a cell is malignant and needs to be killed wherever it's found in the body.

Dr. Sprenger explained, "You need antigen presenting cells. One kind of antigen presenting cell that's potent is dendritic cells, which work like sentinels. We get precursors of dendritic cells from the patient's blood, and in the lab we turn them into dendritic cells and 'load' them with information about the cancer cells. Then we re-inject the dendritic cells (antigen presenting cells) into the patient so they go to the T lymphocytes and introduce this information to them. Then the T lymphocytes go throughout the body and try to encounter the antigens that are only found on tumor cells. This educates the immune system!"

Making the dendritic cells requires a special laboratory of the highest quality, extensive equipment, and a lot of time and man hours. It's a high tech procedure that's unavoidably expensive. It's perfectly safe because the dendritic cells that are injected into the patient are autologous, meaning that they come from the patient's own cells. They're not an alien, unnatural substance.

Unlike the typical holistic or integrative clinic, the IOZK clinic doesn't do much detox. As Dr. Sprenger explained, "What we're doing is so strong and so specific that we focus on the immunotherapy. With our therapy the immune system distinguishes between healthy and unhealthy cells. We teach the immune system to 'go for it.' That's why our patients avoid severe side effects. Patients come here for a couple of hours, and then they can leave and go back to their hotel room. There are no severe side effects, and there's no need to be an in-patient."

The IOZK clinic is unique. Dr. Sprenger said, "We can only administer the therapy here. We have state approval for dendritic cells and also for the Newcastle virus. We're the only clinic in Europe that can legally offer both of these therapies. Nobody else in Europe has the government approval to use this combination. This is spectacular! It took years to get this approval! One other clinic in Germany is approved for dendritic cells, but not in combination with the Newcastle virus. We can't sell dendritic cells to other clinics because of legal restrictions.

"A patient must know that we're legal and state-approved and that our quality standards are high. We've been doing this for about ten years."

What patients at IOZK can expect

Here's how the immunotherapy program works for the typical outpatient. The first set of treatments lasts two weeks and must be done in Cologne. That's how long it takes to analyze the patient's immune system. A blood test reveals what's working and what's not. When the results are in, the doctor makes a schedule for the patient for a combination of three therapies: (1) the Newcastle disease virus therapy, (2) hyperthermia, and (3) dendritic cell vaccination.

After four weeks, the patient comes back to Cologne for about ten days and gets a second vaccination with dendritic cells. Then the doctors analyze the effectiveness of the treatment by testing the immune system. Dr. Sprenger said that testing the effectiveness of the treatment is important to prevent overstimulation, which might have a detrimental effect.

If the treatment is going well, the patient comes back to Cologne in three or four months, and the doctors test again whether the immune system has been educated and is working as it should. Dr. Sprenger said, "If it's not quite good enough, we can do a booster vaccination. The treatment is individualized. There's no fixed schedule for everybody."

What surprises many patients is the lack of side effects. Dr. Sprenger remarked that many patients think "we're not doing anything" because they feel so well throughout the treatment program. They have the notion that if the clinic were really giving them cancer treatments, they would feel rotten. Some patients ask the doctors, "Are you sure you're treating me?" The quality of life for cancer patients at IOZK is far better than for cancer patients who undergo the harsh conventional treatments like chemo and radiation.

The doctors at IOZK have only seen one mild side effect of the Newcastle disease virus. Patients who get this therapy for the very first time can expect a mild fever and mild flu symptoms within 24 hours. It's not a serious medical problem.

Patients on a tight budget may not be able to handle the cost, which is about 30,000 to 40,000 Euros for the first set of treatments with hyperthermia.

The total cost for each patient depends on the schedule of treatment, because every patient gets an individualized schedule. Some people need only two vaccinations in the first year, and maybe they'll need two more after three years. This would involve far less expense than a patient who needs eight vaccinations within the first year.

The clinic does have some American patients who don't mind making several trips to Cologne to get this unique combination of immune-boosting treatments. If the patient can afford it, one option is to stay in Germany for a whole month and get the first two sets of treatments within that month. But patients who have children or a business to run at home usually go home after the first set of treatments and come back four weeks later for the second round of treatments. Three months later they come back again for another followup visit.

Dr. Sprenger said that some patients came to IOZK from Los Angeles, where they had received dendritic cell therapy in a clinical trial. When the trial was over, they were disappointed that they could get no more dendritic cell treatments in Los Angeles. They found out about IOZK through an internet search and went to Germany to continue the dendritic cell program.

The IOZK clinic has had success even with some late stage cancer patients, as mentioned earlier, but it's always better to start the immunotherapy earlier – the earlier the better. Dr. Sprenger said it's best if patients come to the clinic *before* they have their tumor surgically removed so the clinic can get some tumor tissue and use it to prepare the vaccination.

Dr. Sprenger has high praise and deep admiration for the clinic's founder, Dr. Stücker. He said "It's all Dr. Stücker's work. He's an exceptional person. He's a workaholic and a crazy man, and I love him. For more than 15 years he has been consistently working on this, and it was incredibly difficult to get the approval for the Newcastle virus and dendritic cell vaccination. But he did it!"

While patients receive their vaccinations, they get an unexpected benefit. They sit in a chair with an incredible view out the window: Cologne's magnificent Gothic cathedral, one of the greatest works of art ever created by Western civilization. When you tour the cathedral, which is within walking distance of the clinic, it will take your breath away. If you ever have an opportunity to attend an organ recital in the cathedral, do it!

Hotels in Cologne are available to fit any budget, and the clinic is happy to give recommendations for lodging. I stayed at the Hotel Wasserturm (which means water tower). This unique hotel was originally Cologne's water tower and has been converted into a fine place for travelers. Many of the original features have been preserved, including the historic spiral staircase that leads from the ground floor to the next floor. If you stay at the Hotel Wasserturm, you'll also have easy access to the spectacular Agrippa bath, pool, and sauna complex next to the hotel.

Contact information:

IOZK

Hohenstaufenring 30
D-50674 Cologne, Germany

Contact: Dr. Wilfried Stücker, N.D.

Website: IOZK.de

email: info@iozk.de

Phone: 011-49-(0)221-420-399-25

Fax: 011-49-(0)221-420-399-26

Chapter Fourteen

Dr. Marcus Schuermann's clinic in Richterswil, Switzerland

Traditional and complementary medicine meet on the shores of Lake Zurich

Some American doctors suggest a strategy of "watchful waiting" for prostate cancer patients. One of Switzerland's top cancer doctors, Marcus Schuermann, M.D., *totally disagrees*.

When someone has lived with cancer for five or 10 years, the cancer may escape the prostate, resulting in bone metastasis. Instead of ignoring the cancer, Dr. Schuermann says it's better to deal with it and solve the problem.

Dr. Schuermann is the chief physician and oncologist at the ZIO (Zentrum für Integrative Onkologie, which means the Center for Integrative Oncology). The ZIO is located in the town of Richterswil on Switzerland's famous Lake Zurich -- a pristine, crystal clear body of water. This gigantic lake is surrounded by the same kind of Alpine scenery that inspired the famous Rogers & Hammerstein song that begins, "The hills are alive with the sound of music..."

In my opinion, walking by the lakeshore and taking deep breaths of the fresh Swiss air would probably do more good for cancer patients than just about any chemo drug on the market.

Dr. Schuermann has treated patients from all over Germany, Switzerland, Croatia, France, Australia, and a few from America. His cancer treatments are always individualized. If a treatment isn't working, he says that's a clear signal to stop the treatment and try something else.

Dr. Schuermann is a well-informed, open-minded doctor who leans toward conventional medicine while using a remarkable array of natural and holistic therapies. He uses "integrative oncology." He may be just the right cancer doctor for patients who want conventional cancer treatments in combination with natural therapies.

Chemo without the harsh side effects

As a conventionally trained oncologist, Dr. Schuermann uses the tools of classical (conventional) oncology -- surgery, radiation, and chemo -- depending on the case. He integrates classical oncology with hyperthermia, detoxification, nutrition, immune-boosting therapies, oxygenation, exercise, and other therapies.

In some cases, Dr. Schuermann says chemo may be a good idea to reduce the tumor burden. But he gives the chemo in a way that avoids the devastating, unpleasant side-effects of American-style chemo, such as hair-loss, vomiting, and a devastated immune system. To avoid these unwanted side-effects, he doesn't prescribe chemo for three weeks. Instead, he prescribes fractionated chemo, given just one day a week.

In other cases -- melanoma, for example -- Dr. Schuermann says chemo does no good at all. Using chemo in these cases would only enrich the drug companies while ruining the patient's quality of life and hastening his death.

The cheap drug that works *better* than chemo for prostate cancer

When a man has stage four prostate cancer, Dr. Schuermann says no surgery, radiation, or local therapy is effective. In such cases he uses a combination of classical and holistic therapies, including temporary use of a hormone-suppressing medication. He also uses an inexpensive drug he says works much better than chemo: Sitosterol, a synthetic estrogen compound.

Hundreds of patients have used Sitosterol so far, and the results are impressive.

An Australian man took a 12-month supply of Sitosterol with him when he went back home. He had locally advanced prostate cancer, and he's still doing well after two years.

A 70-year-old German man with stage-four prostate cancer was also suffering from bone pain. He chose to use Sitosterol instead of chemo, and his pain went away. When he went off Sitosterol, his PSA started to climb, so he went back on it. His PSA dropped steeply after just three weeks. He would probably still be alive today if he hadn't had such a weak heart: he died a year later because of a diseased heart valve.

Of the hundreds of cancer patients Dr. Schuermann sees every year at the ZIO, most suffer from cancer of the breast or prostate. He also sees some patients with colorectal, ovarian, pancreatic, stomach, and brain cancer.

Cancer patients at the ZIO can get moderate whole body hyperthermia, which takes four hours: one hour to reach the desired core temperature, two hours at the temperature plateau, and one hour to come back down to a normal temperature.

I asked Dr. Schuermann what kind of dietary recommendations he gives cancer patients. He recommends lots of vegetables and fruit.

He doesn't recommend some of the special anti-cancer diets like Budwig, Coy, or Gerson, because, he says, the patient could lose weight on those diets, and that could be a problem.

In addition, he said that some cancer diets, (the Coy diet, for example, which is completely carbohydrate-free) are so strict that it's just about impossible to stay on them for more than a couple of months. Perhaps five percent of patients can do it, he said.

Dr. Schuermann said cancer patients should definitely avoid an excess of sugar and carbohydrates because tumor cells consume large amounts of sugar. When you deprive the tumor cells of fuel, you can get the upper hand against cancer.

His cancer patients go through herbal detoxification therapies to flush toxins out of the liver, kidneys, and muscles. A weekly or twice-weekly infusion of vitamin C by IV detoxifies the muscles.

Colonic hydrotherapy to cleanse the colon is available off-site. In addition, Dr. Schuermann can refer patients who have mercury amalgam dental fillings to a biological dentist who can safely replace them with non-toxic fillings. He sometimes refers patients who have dental problems to the Paracelsus clinic in Lustmühle near St. Gallen. Paracelsus has a state-of-the-art dental clinic.

New computerized therapy helps stressed patients *relax*

For stress management and relaxation, Dr. Schuermann recommends a form of music therapy called HerzMusik (heart music). The patient's own heartbeat, when he or she is in a relaxed state, is converted to musical sounds through a sophisticated computer software program.

Here's how Bernd Orzessek, M.D., one of Switzerland's leading authorities on HerzMusik, explains it: "The data of the heartbeat sequences which we collect during the time of relaxation are analyzed in regard to the musical aspects in it by the means of a specialized software. In the computer, the notes are handed over to all the flutes, violins, harps being transformed into music. You will get an audio CD and you will be able to listen to your heart as often as you like."

Listening to this personalized "heart music" helps put the patient into a relaxed state. This unique therapy is inexpensive. For 150 Swiss francs, a computer converts the sound of your heartbeat into music, and you get a CD of your own HerzMusik. Dr. Schuermann can refer patients to a nearby clinic for this intriguing therapy.

Cancer patients also need to build their lung power. It has been said that deep breathing alone has made many a weak man strong and many a sick man well. Your breath is your power. Deep breathing massages the vital organs and brings revitalizing oxygen into the bloodstream, where it travels throughout the body. Yet many cancer patients are in the unfortunate habit of shallow breathing. They're not getting enough oxygen.

Dr. Schuermann encourages patients to engage in vigorous exercise to build the kind of lung power needed for good health.

As a holistic, integrative physician, Dr. Schuermann recognizes that the three aspects of the patient are body, mind, and spirit. That's why the ZIO also offers art therapy, massage therapy, and counseling. The ZIO also has an operating room, surgeons, urologists, a gastroenterologist, anesthesia, and pain management. The clinic is linked with larger hospitals within nearby Zurich, and Dr. Schuermann attends a weekly tumor board to discuss postoperative treatment suggestions with his colleagues in Zurich.

Dr. Schuermann and his colleagues are leaders in integrative oncology. They sponsor an annual symposium and are organizing a European Society for Integrative Oncology.

Patients find the ZIO a relaxing place to stay, and Dr. Schuermann has an excellent rapport with them. Outpatients can stay at one of the nearby hotels by picturesque Lake Zurich.

Cost of treatment at the ZIO

The foreign exchange rate fluctuates. I will give you the costs in Swiss francs, and you can check the newspaper or the Internet to see what the current exchange rate is. As I write this, the two currencies are close to parity – one Swiss franc buys one dollar.

Costs can change, too. So before you make arrangements to receive treatment in Switzerland, you should get a cost estimate for the proposed treatment plan.

The daily cost for inpatient treatment at the ZIO is 1,500 to 2,000 Swiss francs per day. The outpatient cost is 2,000 to 3,000 francs per week. These prices don't include special diagnostics or prescription medication. They do include low-tech therapies such as vitamin C by IV. Hyperthermia and chemo cost extra.

Each session of local hyperthermia costs 180 francs. Moderate whole body hyperthermia at 39 degrees Celsius costs 500 to 600 francs.

The closest major airport, Zurich, is a 30-minute drive from Richterswil. ZIO also offers integrative oncology in two other places: one in the heart of Zurich and the other in Glarus. I haven't visited either of those branches, but Dr. Schuermann speaks highly of his colleagues there.

Contact information for ZIO:

Dr. Marcus Schuermann

Zentrum für Integrative Onkologie (ZIO)

Bergstraße 16
CH-8805 Richterswil
Switzerland

e-mail: info@integrative-onkologie.ch

Website: www.integrative-onkologie.ch

Phone: 011-41-44-787-27-07

Fax: 011-41-44-787-29-38

Chapter Fifteen

Cancer Dilemma:
Do you swat mosquitoes or drain the swamp?

The typical American cancer doctor focuses on the cancer cells like a laser beam. He makes up his mind to get rid of those cancer cells one way or another, and do "whatever it takes."

Usually step one is to cut the cancer out of the body. And so if the cancer is operable, the tumor is surgically removed.

But everyone knows that a few cancer cells are left behind in the body after surgery. And so to kill off those cells, step two is to burn the cancer cells out of the body by radiation.

And just to make *triple* sure all those cancer cells are gone, step three is to poison any remaining cancer cells with chemotherapy.

The problem is, cancer usually returns. And when it does, then what? More surgery? More radiation? More chemo? After a patient has been run through the wringer of conventional cancer treatments, the return of the cancer is even more devastating than the first diagnosis!

When cancer patients have received their lifetime quota of radiation, they can't have any more of it – even if the cancer returns. As for chemo, sometimes it has no effect on the tumors. The tumors keep growing as if there's no tomorrow, despite massive doses of the most toxic chemotherapies known to man.

Some chemo drugs are effective against one type of cancer, but not another. And frequently doctors – American doctors, at any rate – are just guessing as to whether they're using the right drug for the type of cancer *you* have. There are sophisticated tests to match the drug to the particular cancer cell, but this is another "alternative" approach that few American doctors use.

Sadly, the American approach to cancer treatment ("cut-burn-poison") is all too often a dead end. In other cases it leaves cancer patients disfigured from surgery or sickened or weakened.

If one may compare the cancer cell to another pesky parasite, the mosquito, the American-style cancer treatments are like swatting mosquitoes while ignoring the mosquitoes' breeding ground: the swamp. And that's why it often fails.

Swatting mosquitoes isn't enough. It's necessary to drain the swamp!

Whether you receive conventional cancer treatment, alternative treatment, or a combination of both, if you want to get rid of cancer *for good* so that it *never* returns, you have to get serious about draining the swamp.

The German cancer specialists I interviewed recognize that cancer is never a localized problem. In other words, breast cancer isn't simply a disease of the breast, and prostate cancer isn't simply a disease of the prostate. Rather, cancer is a symptom of a systemic disease of the *whole body* – no matter where the tumor may appear.

Something within the body is producing the cancer cells. When people get cancer, it means that their bodies have become the "swamp" (the breeding ground) that allows the "mosquitoes" (cancer cells) to breed, multiply, and spread out of control.

It's necessary to clean up the body's toxic mess

The German cancer doctors I spoke to told me that a cancer patient's body is loaded with toxic wastes and toxic metals.

Typically a cancer patient's colon is clogged with waste, his blood is thick and sludge-like, his lymphatic system is stagnant, his liver – the body's filter – is jam-packed with toxins, his gall bladder accumulates stones, his kidneys are weak, and so on. Because the cancer patient's organs are usually functioning inefficiently, toxins come into the body faster than the patient can get rid of them.

That has to be reversed. And it can be!

"Draining the swamp" involves a serious detoxification process. A three-week course of treatment at a German cancer clinic can give you a good start at detoxification, but it's *only* a start. You have to continue the detoxification at home. It's an ongoing, lifelong project.

Cleanse the colon

The German doctors I interviewed recognize the necessity of "draining the swamp." That's why they *all* recommended colonic hydrotherapy – a low-tech treatment most American doctors ignore or discourage.

From what I've learned in visiting dozens of cancer clinics and speaking with many alternative cancer doctors, the colon is the center of the "swamp." The services of a professional colonic hydrotherapist are inexpensive, and this therapy is highly recommended.

Change your body from acidic to alkaline

An acidic body welcomes cancer, and cancer cells thrive in an acidic environment. The typical American diet, which is high in meat, high in sugar, and low in fruits and vegetables, contributes to an acidic body.

To change from an acidic body to an alkaline body, you can't eat like the typical American. You must eliminate refined sugar because cancer cells love sugar. If you're fighting cancer, stop feeding it! Cut the cancer cells off from their favorite food.

Switch from a high meat diet to one that has little or no meat. Instead of red meat, choose chicken or fish. Eat lots of fruits and vegetables – organic if possible.

A fresh lemonade morning tonic, which you can use to start your day, can help change your body from acidic to alkaline. Here's the recipe for a lemonade tonic:

Squeeze the juice out of a lemon and add two tablespoons of *authentic* Grade B maple syrup – or an amount that suits your taste. You can use Grade A maple syrup, but don't use any kind of cheap, sugary, artificial maple syrup. Add about 10 to 12 ounces of water and some ground cayenne pepper, and stir well or shake it in a shaker cup. You can start with a pinch of cayenne and gradually work your way up to a half-teaspoon.

The lemonade tonic has other benefits, too. It digests mucus, increases circulation, and stimulates the body to produce the hydrochloric acid necessary for digestion.

Flush your lymphatic system

Toxins sometimes get stuck in your lymphatic system. Unlike your circulatory system, your lymphatic system doesn't have a pump. There are only two ways to flush your lymphatic system: exercise or massage.

The easiest way to flush your lymphatic system through exercise is to get one of those mini-trampolines, called a rebounder, that has a bouncing area about a yard in diameter. You can purchase rebounders at sporting goods stores. Ten minutes of bouncing each day will flush your lymphatic system. You don't have to "get air." In other words, your feet don't have to leave the trampoline. Gentle bouncing is enough to do the job.

Cancer patients who are unable to bounce on a rebounder could get a rebounder chair – which would make it much easier but just as effective. You can get more information about rebounder chairs on the Internet at www. BounceBackChairs.com. Another option is to get lymphatic massages from a professional massage therapist.

Help your largest organ – your skin – eliminate waste and renew itself

Sweating is good because it helps your body get rid of toxins through your skin, which is your body's largest organ. Taking a hot sauna and finishing it with a cold shower helps do this.

But an even more effective sauna is the far infrared sauna, which quickly and easily pulls out toxins from deep within the skin. This kind of sauna can even be installed in your home.

Another technique for assisting your skin is dry skin brushing: using no water, you brush every square inch of your skin with a natural bristle brush every day. Why? Because there are several benefits: it cleans pores, exfoliates the skin, keeps skin toned and soft, aids blood circulation, and helps eliminate toxins. Dry skin brushing also stimulates all of your body's acupuncture points, which helps energize the body.

Listen to what the legendary natural healer Dr. Bernard Jensen said about dry skin brushing:

"I believe skin brushing is one of the finest of all baths. No soap can wash the skin as clean as the new skin you have under the old. You make new skin every 24 hours on the body. The skin will be as clean as the blood is. Skin brushing removes the top layer. This helps to eliminate uric acid crystals, catarrh, and various other acids in the body. The skin should eliminate two pounds of waste acids daily. Keep the skin active."

You'll need two different brushes for dry skin brushing: a body brush with a removable handle and a complexion brush. They are available on the Internet from Bernard Jensen Products in Solana Beach, CA 92075. You can get both brushes (the "Skin Care Combo Pack") for less than $20 online at www.bernardjensen.org.

Overlooked secret of surviving cancer: Get rid of the false, negative programming in your mind

An often-overlooked part of the "swamp" is the mind. It's necessary to detoxify the mind by getting rid of the false, negative thoughts and fears that feed cancer. Toxic thinking should be replaced with healing thoughts that kick your immune system into high gear.

Most of the German clinics we visited help the patient focus on this very task. And this is something you can also do at home.

Believe it or not, counseling techniques that change the cancer patient's thought patterns have turned around "hopeless" and "terminal" cases of cancer. It's not just a matter of changing from "negative thinking" to "positive thinking" – though that's part of it. More importantly, it's a matter of changing *false* thinking to *true* thinking.

For example, many if not most cancer patients believe cancer is a powerful, almost invincible enemy, like a juggernaut that's going to crush them. But the late Dr. O. Carl Simonton, M.D., pointed out that the truth is quite different: cancer cells are, in fact, weak, abnormal, and deformed.

Dr. Simonton, a remarkable pioneer in cancer treatment, created a groundbreaking method that helps cancer patients visualize their immune systems vanquishing the weak, deformed cancer cells. His approach is validated by published studies and clinical experience.

To learn more about Dr. Simonton's powerful methods, see the website: www. simontoncenter.com. For just $75 you can order Dr. Simonton's "patient package" from his website. Or you could check out one of his books from your public library and get started with healing thoughts for free.

Other good ways to keep cancer from coming back

It's important to keep your liver, gall bladder, and kidneys working efficiently. You can do that by flushing them once or more a year. Although information about these flushes is available on the Internet, it's much better to find an experienced naturopathic or holistic health practitioner who can guide you in this important area.

A long-term brain cancer survivor from America who got rid of his cancer at a clinic in Germany over five years ago continues to get an intravenous vitamin C infusion every month here in America. Monthly IV infusions of vitamin C seem like a wise idea, and the brain cancer survivor credits them for his continued good health.

German physicians and scientists pioneered enzyme therapy, which all of the German cancer clinics recommend. Enzyme therapy can help prevent cancer from coming back. To get more enzymes, increase your intake of raw fruits and vegetables. You can also get enzyme supplements such as the German product Wobenzym. My publisher offers an excellent introduction to enzyme therapy called *The Missing Ingredient for Good Health*. You can get more information about it at www. CancerDefeated.com.

Magnetic field therapy is another affordable and beneficial therapy you can use in your home as part of the strategy to keep cancer from coming back.

Chapter Sixteen

How to raise funds or get insurance reimbursement for your cancer treatment in Germany

The cost of cancer treatment in Germany might run about $35,000, more or less, depending on where you go, how long you stay at the clinic or hospital, and what treatments you get. The cost of getting rid of prostate cancer through transurethral local hyperthermia is less than $10,000. Certainly the cost is a bargain, compared to the six-figure price tag at American clinics and hospitals – typically $350,000 to $1,000,000!

Furthermore, German cancer clinics can also boast an impressive record of success: when American cancer doctors give up on their cancer patients, Germany's top doctors stand ready to use milder, more effective methods to cure the cancer. And they often succeed – even in "hopeless" and "terminal" cases.

Still, it can be tough to scrape together an extra $35,000 – roughly the price of a new mini-van.

One option is to obtain a loan. A company called Med Loan Finance, based in Kansas, has helped many patients get financing for medical treatment outside the United States. To get an application, you can call their toll-free number or visit their website. You'll find their contact information below.

If you have a life insurance policy (term or whole), you may be able to borrow against your policy from Life Credit Company, which offers "living benefit loans" for medical expenses. Through this company you could get a cash advance of up to half of the value of your life insurance policy to pay for alternative cancer treatment, collateralized by the life insurance.

This kind of loan enables financially stressed cancer patients to pay for the integrative, holistic treatment that's most likely to be successful, instead of choosing conventional cancer treatment because that's what's covered by the health insurance policy.

The best outcome financially, of course, is to get insurance reimbursement for your cancer treatment in Germany. There's no guarantee that you'll get reimbursed. But if you have health insurance, there's a good chance that you can get some or most of your expenses reimbursed. Don't count on being reimbursed, but it's certainly worth filing a claim!

There's a company that will negotiate with your insurance company on your behalf to help you obtain reimbursement. It's called American Medical Health Alliance, and it's based in Houston, Texas. American Medical Health Alliance gets a percentage of the reimbursement as compensation for their services, and that gives them a strong incentive to get you as much reimbursement as possible. The more you get, the more they make. It's a win/win deal.

Many cancer patients have successfully raised funds for their alternative cancer treatment through a crowdfunding and fundraising website such as www.GoFundMe.com or www.YouCaring.com. One cancer patient who successfully raised funds through YouCaring chose that website because "they don't charge the processing fees that GoFundMe does."

Contact information:

Med Loan Finance (for financing)

10515 W 148th Terrace
Overland Park, KS 66221

Phone: 800-504-4053

Fax: 800-555-8122

e-mail: info@MedLoanFinance.com

Website: www.MedLoanFinance.com

Life Credit Company (for financing)

7911 Herschel Avenue, Suite 201
La Jolla, CA 92037

Phone: 888-274-1777

Website: www.LifeCreditCompany.com

American Medical Health Alliance
(for insurance reimbursement)

11807 Westheimer Road #550-158
Houston, TX 77077

Phone: 800-221-0817

Fax: 281-580-1453

e-mail: info@amhabilling.com

Website: www.amhabilling.com

Crowdfunding and fundraising websites:

www.YouCaring.com
www.GoFundMe.com

Endnote

How to find the German clinic that's right for you

When I talk about the "German clinics," I don't mean to exclude the fine clinics in Switzerland and Austria. Rather, I use the expression "German clinics" in a broad sense to encompass the complementary cancer clinics in all German-speaking lands.

People have asked me, "If you had cancer, which clinic would you choose?" That's a good question. I don't have cancer, and I hope I never get it. I don't know which clinic I would choose. All of the clinics and doctors featured in this book impress me. They use an integrative approach – a combination of natural medicine and conventional medicine. Whether you prefer a clinic that tilts toward the side of natural medicine or a clinic that tilts the other way, you'll probably find at least one clinic in this book that suits your preference.

The choice of a clinic depends on many factors, including what kind of cancer a patient has and how far advanced it is. If you have cancer, and if you're considering the possibility of going to a German clinic for treatment, I'm sure you'll read each chapter in this book carefully. After reading the book, you may feel drawn to a particular clinic. If you find that three clinics stand out as strong choices, of course you'll have to narrow it down to one.

Perhaps the easiest way to find the German cancer clinic that's right for you is to seek the advice of an independent medical advisor. The advisor I recommend without hesitation is Dr. Adem Günes, M.D., Ph.D. Dr. Günes was the right-hand-man of Dr. Frank Daudert, and he has vast experience not only as a cancer doctor but also as a medical researcher.

Most recently Dr. Günes has been hired to establish cancer clinics in Thailand that meet the high standards of the cancer clinics in Germany and provide the same integrative treatment protocols.

I was surprised to learn that the government of Thailand formally recognizes and supports alternative medicine. Thailand is the only country in the world that has two health ministers – one for conventional medicine and the other for alternative medicine.

I haven't visited the cancer clinics in Thailand, but Lothar Hirneise, the founder of the 3E Center near Stuttgart, told me, "In medicine, Thailand is far superior to just about every other country. The way they handle you, you're a king in the hospital. The hospitals are like five star hotels. They do outstanding work." I'm pleased to know that Dr. Günes is involved is establishing the Thai cancer clinics.

If there is a man who knows more about natural medicine than Dr. Günes, I would like to meet him. He is one of the most brilliant German doctors I have ever met. To find out more about Dr. Günes's services as an independent medical advisor, log onto his website www.dr-adem.com. You may send Dr. Günes an e-mail at this address: contact@dr-adem.com.

A few Americans who get rid of their cancer in Germany can afford to return to Germany again and again for follow-up care, but most cannot. In the current edition of this book, I have included information about how to find a cooperative, open-minded American doctor who can give you the long-term follow-up care you need to keep cancer from coming back.

Be prepared to make permanent lifestyle changes. You should certainly avoid junk food, processed food, and sugar, you should exercise – at least a daily half-hour walk – and you may want to incorporate the German-recommended Budwig protocol in your daily eating plan.

Many people found the earlier editions of this book helpful, and I got positive customer feedback from readers who actually went to Germany for cancer treatment. If you or a loved one have cancer, my hope and prayer is that you'll find this book helpful.

If you liked this book...

If you liked this book, perhaps you might like Andrew Scholberg's other books about cancer clinics and alternative treatments.

Amish Cancer Secret: How to cure just about any cancer the Amish way by Frank Cousineau with Andrew Scholberg is a book about the top alternative cancer clinics in Mexico. If you're interested, see this website: www.CancerDefeated.com.

America's Best Cancer Doctors and Their Secrets by Frank Cousineau with Andrew Scholberg is a book about the top alternative cancer clinics in America. If you're interested, see this website: www.CancerDefeated.com.

How to Cure Almost Any Cancer at Home for $5.15 a Day by Bill Henderson with Andrew Scholberg describes the seven-point Bill Henderson Protocol to whip just about any cancer at home. If you're interested, see this website: www.CancerDefeated.com.

The 31 Day Home Cancer Cure by Ty Bollinger with Andrew Scholberg describes Ty Bollinger's home protocol that's so effective that a terminal hospice patient in Louisiana who used it was able to check out of the hospice – not by going to the cemetery but by going home to enjoy some bonus years! If you're interested, see this website: www.CancerDefeated.com.